Breastfeeding Your Baby

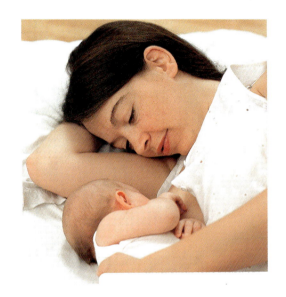

CW01151297

Heather Welford

MARSHALL PUBLISHING • LONDON

A Marshall Edition
Conceived, edited and designed by
Marshall Editions
161 New Bond Street, London WIY 9PA

First published in the UK in 2000 by
Marshall Publishing Ltd

ISBN: 184028 290 8

Originated in Singapore by Chroma Graphics
Printed and bound in China by Excel Printing

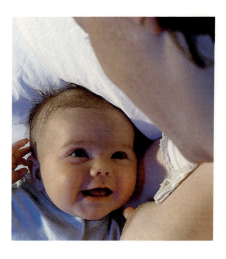

Project Editor Gwen Rigby

Art Editor Frances de Rees

Picture Research Elizabeth Loving

Managing Editor Anne Yelland

Managing Art Editor Helen Spencer

Editorial Director Ellen Dupont

Art Director Dave Goodman

Editorial Coordinator Becca Clunes

Production Amanda Mackie

Note

Every effort has been taken to make sure that
all information in this book is correct and
compatible with national standards generally
accepted at the time of publication. This book is
not intended to replace consultation with your
doctor or other healthcare professional. The
author and publisher disclaim any liability, loss,
injury, or damage incurred as a consequence,
directly or indirectly, of the use and application
of the contents of this book.

CONTENTS

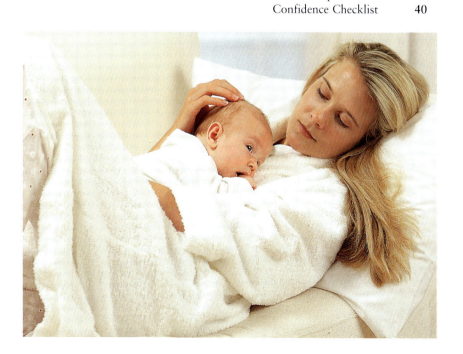

Everyday Breastfeeding

Solving Breastfeeding Problems

Breastfeeding an Older Baby

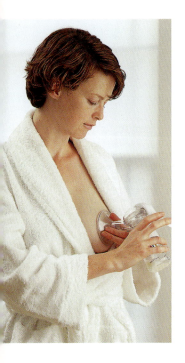

Special Situations

INTRODUCTION

So you're planning on breastfeeding your baby? Or maybe you've started to breastfeed, and want to know about how it may change as time goes on? Do you have problems, and want to know how to overcome them? Or perhaps you're undecided about feeding, and not sure if breastfeeding will work out well for you and your baby? Whatever your questions, and your plans, this book will help you.

There's no doubt at all that breastfeeding is the healthy choice for both you and your baby. As we'll see, there are numerous, proven health benefits for you as a woman, and for your baby, both now and in the future. Artificial feeding, sometimes known as formula feeding, can never have the same nutritional profile of breastfeeding.

A NATURAL ACTIVITY

The psychological and emotional experience you share with your baby when you feed him from your own body is one that most mothers feel is very special and worthwhile. When it's going well, breastfeeding is rewarding and fulfilling, an experience which many mothers remember with joy and

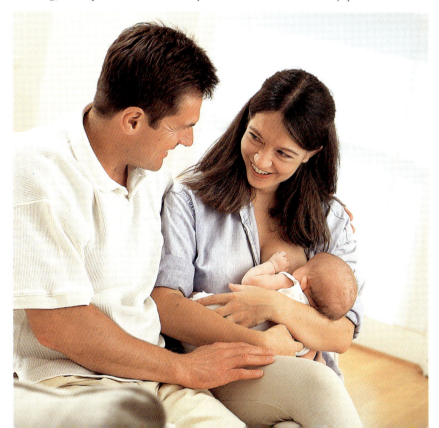

satisfaction. It is also the natural way to feed infants. Right from the moment of conception, your body simply assumes that you will breastfeed. The breasts respond to pregnancy hormones by beginning a process of laying down new milk-producing and milk-storing tissue, and blood and lymph vessels. This is sometimes felt as a tingling sensation in the breasts.

The Montgomery's tubercles – tiny sebaceous glands on the areola, the dark area around the nipple – become more prominent as they prepare to keep the nipples soft and supple. In fact, these breast changes begin early in pregnancy. They may be enough to make you suspect you're pregnant – even before you've missed your first period.

Later in pregnancy, your breasts will enlarge, and you may notice some leaking of colostrum, the highly nutritious fluid the breasts make for your baby to have in the first days after the birth. Even if you never put him to the breast, you will make milk. So, everything is in place without you are making a decision about feeding – it's truly natural.

STARTING TO BREASTFEED

A healthy, full-term baby has a powerful sucking and swallowing reflex, which allows him to come on to the breast and begin feeding immediately after the birth. He also has a 'rooting' reflex – he moves his head and mouth showing that he's actively seeking the breast and looking for food.

That's not to say the process of feeding and of making breastfeeding a happy and fulfilling activity happens without any hitch. It may be natural, but the skills involved don't come naturally to every mother and baby pair. Every mother, and every baby, must learn to breastfeed. For some, the learning takes place within seconds – almost literally straightaway both get the hang of breastfeeding without a problem. But it's fair to say that this smooth transition to breastfeeding is probably a minority experience. For most of us, it's more of a challenge. Why should it be that way? Why would nature have made it anything other than simple to do? The fact is that many things interfere with the establishment of easy, happy breastfeeding.

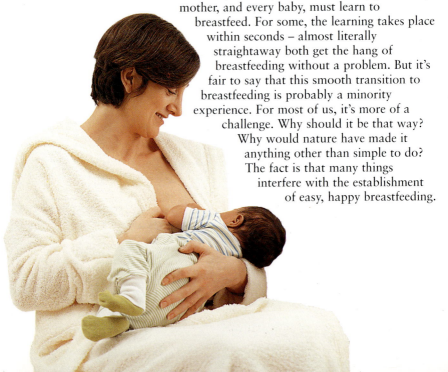

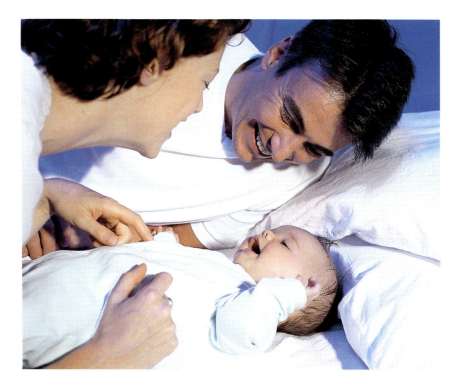

Here are some of them.

■ A baby who's born pre-term may not have well-developed reflexes.

■ Medical treatment for mother or baby after the birth may delay the start of breastfeeding.

■ Some pain-relieving drugs used during labour may make the baby sleepy and unresponsive.

■ Lack of help with positioning the baby comfortably may make breastfeeding painful.

■ Few women have seen babies being breastfed, and this makes it harder for them to know what the best position is for effective breastfeeding.

■ Breastfeeding may be regarded as difficult, and this negative attitude affects a mother's confidence.

■ Lack of good, consistent information about breastfeeding can lead the mother to be confused.

■ Lack of support and encouragement can mean that the mother loses heart.

■ Hospital practices that actively work against breastfeeding (such as separating mother and baby) can make it more difficult to get it going.

■ Ideas about baby care that favour routine and predictability work against breastfeeding.

More rarely, there may be physical or other problems that affect breastfeeding. Babies who are born with a cleft lip and/or palate, for example, may not be able to suck at the breast at all, although there are sometimes solutions to this problem. And mothers who have truly inverted nipples may need extra help in getting the baby latched on.

Sometimes, breastfeeding doesn't start smoothly for reasons we don't fully understand, and it can be hard to keep on breastfeeding when your baby is difficult to feed or cries a lot. It can even feel like rejection. We'll discuss these feelings, and these difficulties – common and not so common – in this book.

ENCOURAGING BREASTFEEDING

With the greater availability of breast milk substitutes and the bottles to contain them, breastfeeding has declined throughout this century. More recently, though, we've learned just how valuable breastfeeding can be – and the decline seems to have been arrested and even reversed.

However, the problem remains that some of the skills surrounding breastfeeding have skipped a generation or more, and many mothers today find their own mothers and grandmothers are poorly informed about breastfeeding and are unable to give much support. Many health professionals, too, are not trained in helping mothers establish breastfeeding.

On the plus side, we've seen the growth of mother-to-mother networks, which help by spreading accurate information, and by giving friendly, encouraging support when it's needed.

Books like this one also help to fill the information gap – and offer you support and affirmation that what you're doing is wonderful for your baby, rewarding for you, and worthwhile for your family.

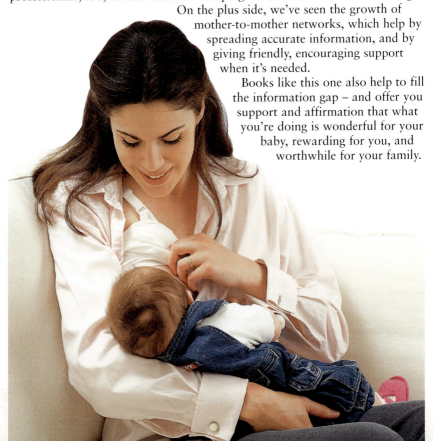

CHOOSING TO BREASTFEED

Mothers have breastfed their babies for some 30,000 generations. Now, for the first time, alternatives to breast milk are widely and cheaply available, but most mothers still choose to breastfeed – at least initially – because they feel it is best.

Feeding your baby at the breast isn't just a way of giving him a healthy, nourishing start in life. It's a warm, loving and hugely enjoyable way to get close to him, and for him to feel secure, safe and cared for.

In this chapter we show you how making that choice gives your baby several health and developmental advantages, and how it impacts on your own health. We give practical information and answer some of the questions women ask about how breastfeeding will affect them.

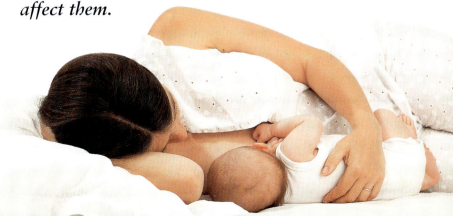

A HEALTHY START

Breastfeeding gives human babies the milk that's meant for them. Other milks commonly given to babies are based on cow's milk – or sometimes on milk from goats or the soya bean – and they're often known as 'formula'. It sounds scientific and, indeed, the milk has to be altered considerably before it is safe for a new baby's digestive system.

But while the milk is modified according to a 'recipe', it can't begin to be the same as breast milk. We humans produce our own 'species specific' milk – the milk that has evolved to suit the growth and development of our own young. Other mammals' milk is different, and while it's perfect for their young, it can't be as ideally suited to ours.

Indeed, if breastfeeding has special advantages, giving formula milk has disadvantages. If breastfeeding protects a baby from certain illnesses and conditions, bottle feeding carries risks that the baby may be affected by them. So, to breastfeed is to avoid unnecessary risk.

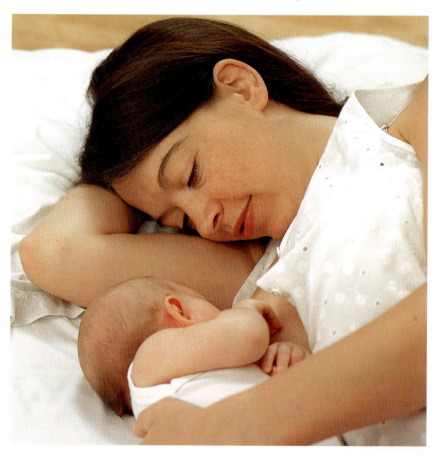

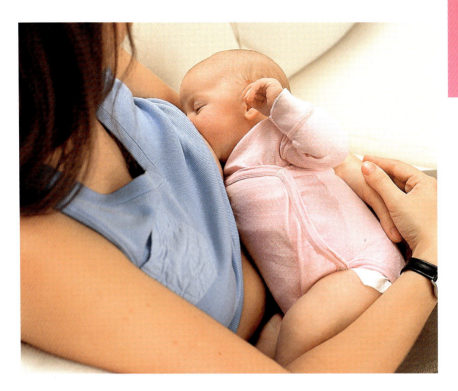

HOW BREAST MILK DIFFERS FROM FORMULA

The proportions of the ingredients in breast milk are different from those in formula – for instance, there is about twice as much protein in cow's milk formula as there is in breast milk. The ratio of the ingredients is very different, too – breast milk has a higher proportion of polyunsaturated fatty acids, compared with formula.

There are many ingredients in breast milk that are not present at all in formula, or are present in only tiny amounts. Breast milk contains immunoglobulins; phagocytes; T lymphocytes; enzymes such as lysozymes; and many other substances that help to protect the infant against infections, as well as cells, antibodies, hormones and other important constituents. Where manufacturers have added some constituents to some brands of formula, they are not from human sources, so they cannot be identical.

But even though we can be sure that the ingredients of breast milk are there in the right quantities for baby humans – just as we can be sure that otter's milk is right for baby otters, cat's milk is right for kittens, and cow's milk is perfect for calves – there is a further important difference.

Breast milk is a living fluid, changing and responding to the needs of the baby as he grows and develops. It contains important anti-infective ingredients that help the baby fight infection and disease and, most amazingly, it can make an instant response to infection by producing a whole new set of powerful immunoglobulins that boost the baby's immune system by fighting off bacteria and viruses.

HOW BREASTFEEDING PROTECTS A BABY

When the mother comes into contact with a disease-causing organism – as all of us do, every day – it enters her body via her respiratory system or her gastro-intestinal system. In response, the mucous membrane lining her lungs and her gut produce an immune response, which protects her and which also enters the bloodstream. The immunoglobulins thus produced travel to the breasts and enter the breast milk in a form that can be processed by the baby the next time he comes to the breast; so protecting him in the same way that his mother is protected.

This is really important, since babies are born with very immature immune systems, and the actual and potential protection given by breast milk fills that immunity gap.

Babies fed on formula are missing out on the protection offered by breast milk. In addition, great care must be taken when preparing their feeds and sterilizing bottles and teats, which can easily harbour bacteria if they're not scrupulously clean. It's also why it makes sense for babies to be kept close to their mothers, especially in the early days and weeks, in order to make the most of this wonderful immune response.

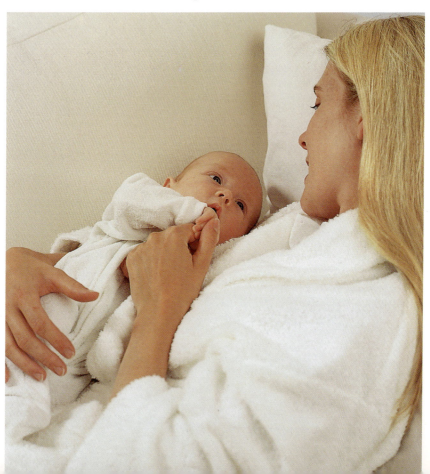

THE PROTECTION BREASTFED BABIES RECEIVE

Research with large numbers of babies in different environments, including the industrialized cities of the West, has shown that breastfed babies are less likely to suffer from:

- gastroenteritis
- respiratory infections
- ear infections
- urinary infections
- allergies
- asthma
- eczema

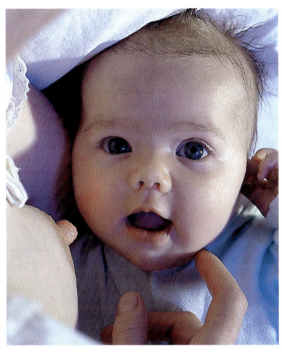

In the studies that accurately demonstrate the benefits of breastfeeding, a control has been set up to monitor the social and economic background of the babies in the study. Otherwise, it could be concluded that it is something connected with the lives of breastfed babies or their parents that makes them healthier, rather than the fact that they're breastfed. Many such studies have been done, and they show conclusively that it is breastfeeding that makes the difference, and nothing else.

THE MORE, THE BETTER

There is good evidence for what doctors call a 'dose related response', too. That means, the more breastfeeding, the better. So, while some studies show that even one feed at the breast seems to give the baby some protection, it is worthwhile continuing for a longer time. There is no magic cut-off point for stopping breastfeeding – breast milk is always healthy and nourishing – and many mothers and babies carry on for a long time, alongside other foods and drinks, just because they like it.

In the West, many of the conditions, such as gastroenteritis or ear infections, that breastfeeding guards against are not normally life threatening, as they may be in the developing world. But it is always distressing for a baby to suffer from vomiting and diarrhoea, and it is very stressful to care for a miserable baby crying in pain from an ear infection. If they become really ill, babies may even have to be hospitalized as a result of these conditions, which is upsetting and disturbing for the whole family.

THE LASTING BENEFITS

Breastfeeding is not just good for your baby while he's very young, or for as long as he is breastfed and having no other food or drink. It appears to alter the immune system and to have lasting, positive effects on health and on intelligence.

For example, in one project, breastfeeding without any formula milk or solid foods to 15 weeks has been shown to have measurable benefits with regard to respiratory infection up to the age of at least seven years (the age at which the children were studied).

Some breastfeeding (with or without the addition of formula) to 13 weeks offers significant long-term protection against gastroenteritis up to the age of 18 months to 2 years.

It may be that these benefits have longer-lasting effects – and at least one major programme is looking at infant feeding with reference to the health of 13-year-olds. By following the same group of babies all the way through their childhood years, and even into adulthood, it should be possible to say more precisely in what ways, and for how long, breastfeeding matters.

There is speculation that it may reduce the risk of heart disease developing. Breastfeeding may even help to prevent obesity. We already know that childhood onset diabetes is less common in babies who are breastfed; it could be that adult diabetics are also more likely to have been bottle fed.

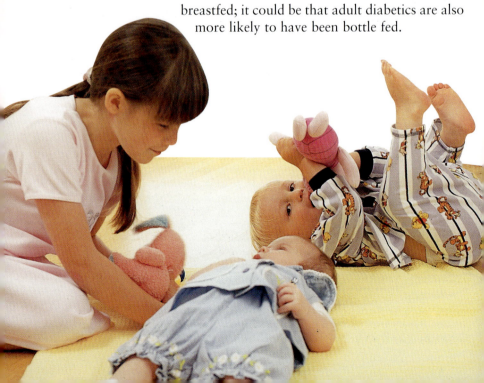

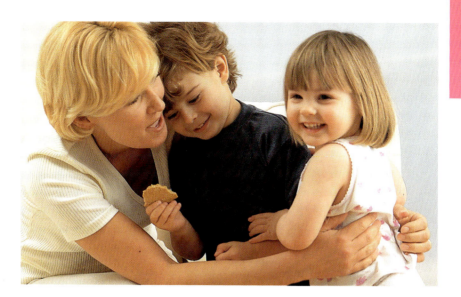

CAN BREASTFEEDING AFFECT INTELLIGENCE?

There is some evidence that breastfed babies are smarter than bottle-fed babies, although measuring intelligence is one of the more difficult tasks in medical research. Is it the act of breastfeeding that promotes the development of intelligence – the way eye contact is established, and the interaction between mother and baby? Or is it the ingredients in breast milk?

Some studies looked at pre-term babies who were fed milk by tube, so they looked at the 'ingredients' factor rather than the 'interaction' factor. Of course, a control is needed for all social and hereditary factors. If it were only parents with IQs of 150-plus who breastfed, we would not be amazed if their children were also very intelligent. However, in all reputable studies, breastfed babies – whether they have been tube fed or breastfed directly – tend to outperform babies who have been formula fed.

It seems likely that the ingredients in breast milk are partly responsible for higher intelligence, and also possible that it results from the interaction of mother and baby.

WHY BREASTMILK IS SO BENEFICIAL

At birth, your baby's brain is relatively small, but during the first two years of life the brain undergoes more growth than it ever will again. Breast milk has a hugely complex arrangement of long-chain unsaturated fatty acids (LCPs), which are known to be vitally important in the development and growth of the infant brain, especially the areas we know to be associated with intelligence. LCPs are now added to some brands of formula milk during processing, and some studies show that they make a difference (other studies have, however, shown no effect). Since these LCPs come from non-human sources, they cannot be identical to those in breast milk and, as a result, their function is likely to be different.

BENEFITS FOR MOTHERS

As we've seen, breastfeeding is, and has been, the usual way to feed a baby, since humankind began to evolve.

All the changes in your breasts that you experienced at puberty took place in preparation for breastfeeding, and during pregnancy and after the birth, your body 'assumes' that this is what you're going to do (see pages 20–21).

Using your breasts to feed your baby is, therefore, a natural thing for you to do, and it appears, from the research, to bring some lasting protective benefits to mothers as well as babies.

PRE-TERM AND SICK BABIES NEED YOUR BREASTMILK

Small, vulnerable, pre-term and sick babies need breast milk, too. Even if you can't feed your baby directly at the breast, you can stay in touch with him by expressing milk for him to have by tube, cup or bottle. This can be an important link that helps you get close to your baby, and helps *you* through this more difficult transition to parenthood. You are doing something that makes you feel good about yourself and your baby. For more information on the practicalities of feeding in this way, see pages 98–99 and 102–103.

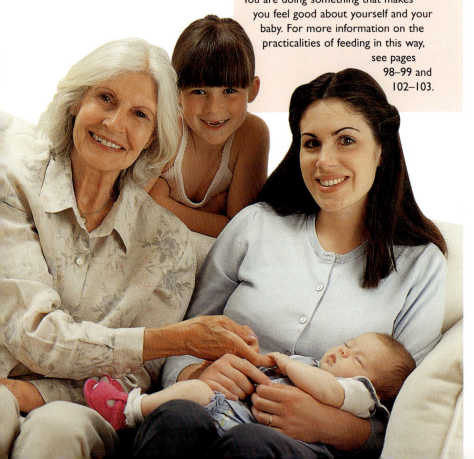

HOW BREASTFEEDING HELPS WOMEN

Breastfeeding has hormonal effects on the body which may offer protection from certain conditions in later life. Not breastfeeding, or not breastfeeding for a long period, could mean that the optimum hormonal profile isn't achieved – laying women open to the risk of disease. Women who breastfeed:

■ are less likely to develop pre-menopausal breast cancer, and it seems that the longer you breastfeed the better – total up the time if you have more than one child.

■ are less likely to develop ovarian cancer.

■ are less likely to suffer fractures in middle and old age (common as a result of osteoporosis, the bone disease that can affect older women).

MOTHERS ENJOY BREASTFEEDING, TOO!

Breastfeeding releases endorphins – natural mood-enhancing and soothing substances – into the bloodstream, and when it's going well, many women report that the act of breastfeeding is very relaxing. That's not to say you'll be so laid back that you're lethargic and even sleepy. Far from it. The subtle feeling of good humour is probably there so that mothers enjoy breastfeeding – nature's way of ensuring that you get pleasure out of it and are therefore more likely to carry on with it.

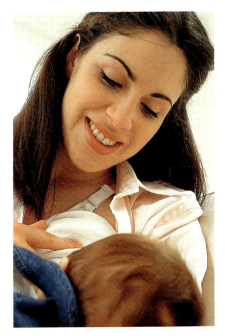

In addition, seeing your baby thrive on your milk is enormously satisfying. Mothers often say they feel proud of themselves, and feel that by breastfeeding their babies they have achieved something special and unique.

From very early on, babies show in many ways how much they enjoy the warmth, security and closeness of breastfeeding. The expression of enjoyment ranges from the young baby who comes off the breast full and satisfied, with an expression of drunken contentment on his face, to the older baby who wriggles with glee when he sees a feed is coming, and the frightened toddler who finds the fears of a bad dream go away when he's soothed at the breast.

In addition, you know you are offering something that's more than just top-quality milk when you're breastfeeding. This makes you feel good – and why not? Breastfeeding is, after all, the one thing you, as a mother, can do for your baby that no one else can.

EASY BREASTFEEDING

Is breastfeeding a tie? Is it something that means your life as a new parent is awkward and more demanding than it needs to be? Does breastfeeding just mean more hard work that no one can help you with?

Babies are, of course, a tie in themselves – and they tend to be that way for at least 20 years or so. Your child's needs, and your child's future, will always have to figure in your plans, whether you're thinking about tomorrow, next week, next month or even the next decade or so.

YOUR BABY'S READY MEAL

Your breast milk is there, on tap, always ready at just the right temperature for your baby – away from home, while travelling, while visiting. That's a lot more convenient than having to carry bottles and formula and worrying about kettles and cleanliness wherever you go!

When people say that breastfeeding is a tie, they mean that you always have to be with your baby, and you can't share the care with someone else. The idea is that this will stop you enjoying yourself or pursuing your own interests – because the places you can be with a baby, or the places you'd want to take your baby to, are restricted. This is true, but only in a very limited way.

BREASTFEEDING CAN BE SIMPLE

Here are some facts to reassure you, and those people around you, who raise doubts about breastfeeding.

■ Small babies are very portable and, while young, there are few places they can't be taken quite easily.

■ If you need to be away from your baby, you can leave expressed breast milk (see pages 58–59), and you can plan your day so that after the newborn period you can have occasional short spells away from him between feeds.

■ Your baby needs breast milk alone for a very short time indeed – four to six months. The rest of the 18–20 years of parental care he'll be increasingly less dependent on your constant presence.

ISN'T BREASTFEEDING HARD WORK?

Look at the work of breastfeeding a baby – when you can sit or lie down, or do something else one-handed – next to the comparatively heavy-duty tasks of:

■ washing bottles, teats and other feeding accessories

■ rinsing them

■ sterilizing them

■ making up the feeds

■ heating up the feed when it's needed

■ washing extra baby clothes (because sicked-up baby formula is smelly – unlike breast milk, which can be wiped away leaving no smell)

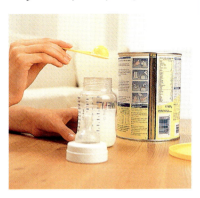

The idea that no one else can help you with baby care if you're breastfeeding is wrong. There are many tasks to share with your partner, or to delegate to him, and they are not all chores such as cooking, washing and ironing. For instance, bathtime and nappy changing are ways in which fathers can get to know their baby and to give him physical care and plenty of interaction – (The nappy of a breastfed baby is a lot less smelly than that of a bottle-fed baby.)

A young baby needs a great deal of cuddling and soothing, and this doesn't have to come just as part of feeding. Partners, and other family members, can get close to your baby in this way and give you a break at the same time. Your baby will gradually learn that love comes in many forms, and it doesn't have to come accompanied by food and drink.

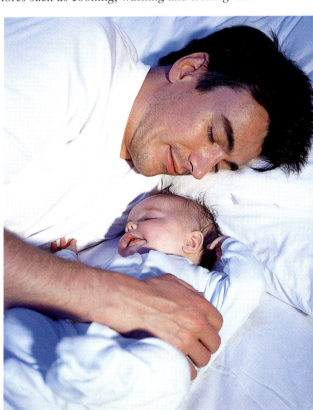

GETTING READY

One of the first signs you're pregnant may well be changes in your breasts. The hormonal changes associated with conception have an almost immediate effect on your breasts. There is an increased blood supply to your breasts, and they start, very gradually, to lay down milk-producing and milk-storing tissue.

SIGNS OF PREGNANCY

Some women notice one or more of these signs even before they've missed their first menstrual period.

■ The nipples and their surrounding areolae may look a little darker in colour.

■ The breasts are more sensitive, even tender.

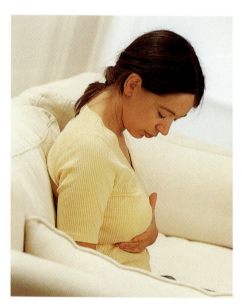

■ The Montgomery's tubercles, which look like small spots on the nipples, become more prominent. These are actually the exit points of tiny sebaceous glands that secrete a fluid to soften the skin of the breasts and keep it supple.

Later on, as pregnancy progresses, the breasts may feel larger and firmer than they've been before. The nipples and areolae tend to darken as the pigment that gives them their colour deepens. The shape of the nipples may change a little as well: flattish nipples tend to stand out more. Some women leak colostrum from their nipples in the last weeks or months of pregnancy. This is nothing to be concerned about.

CARING FOR YOUR BREASTS DURING PREGNANCY

You may be given advice to 'toughen the nipples' with brisk towel rubs, but there's no evidence that this preparation is necessary, and it could even be uncomfortable.

If you leak colostrum, you could wear breast pads (bought from the chemist) for convenience, but most women find they don't need to bother.

If colostrum dries on your nipples, warm water will take it off. Avoid cleaning your nipples with soap – it can be drying, and may remove the natural sebum that's there to moisturize your skin.

WHAT ABOUT BRAS?

There's no magic about a bra – it's there to keep you comfortable, that's all, and some women feel they look a better shape in one. If you want to wear one, do so, and get one that fits to ensure your comfort.

It's probably a good idea to buy a special bra when you are about seven to eight months pregnant, since your breasts are unlikely to get much larger from that point on, and you may not want to spend time shopping later. Most nursing or maternity bras have a fastening and straps that will adjust to give you an extra inch or so if you need it after the baby's born, and they will allow you to adjust it later when you may not need quite so much room.

BEING FITTED

You need to try on several bras before you decide which one to buy. Make sure that the straps don't dig into your shoulders and that the back fastening doesn't ride up.

Try fastening and unfastening the cups with one hand – is it easy? Whether you go for a drop cup, a front fastening, or zippered cups is your preference. Just make sure nothing presses on your flesh, since this is thought to be a possible cause of a blocked duct (see pages 68–69).

If you're fairly small- to medium-breasted, you can get away with a normal bra. When it comes to feeding, you can bring one breast out of the top at a time. But, once again, make sure that nothing presses into your breasts.

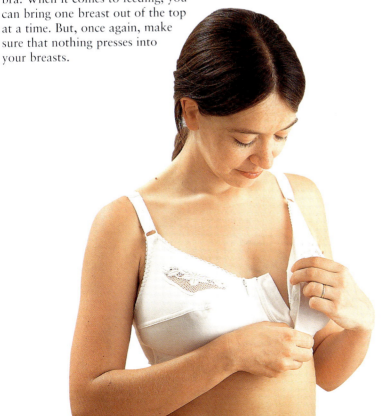

CONFIDENCE CHECKLIST

If breastfeeding is new to you, here's what you can do to build up your confidence, which will help you make a success of it.

- Read about breastfeeding, and learn as much about it as you can.

- Talk to other breastfeeding mothers.

- Join a group of mothers or parents, and make new friends who'll be supportive to you.

- Ask about breastfeeding at your antenatal class.

- Talk to a midwife about your anxieties, and raise any questions you may have with her.

- Find out from female relatives what they experienced – it may be negative, and if it was, find out why.

- Some areas have special classes about breastfeeding for pregnant women. Ask your midwife about them.

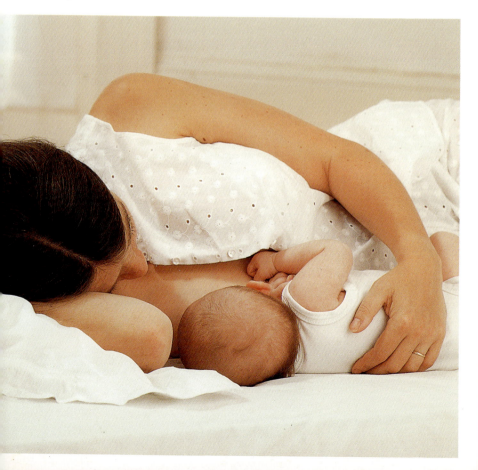

THE EARLY DAYS

Breastfeeding is a learning experience, and for some mothers, and some babies, a time of setbacks and challenges. For others, the process gets under way easily and smoothly. Having a baby is an emotional time, feeding problems can seem overwhelming, and you can feel very stressed and inadequate if you think you're not getting things right.

Most breastfeeding difficulties are temporary, and they do have a solution. There are many ways in which you can help yourself and your baby, and the professionals should give you the information and support you need to breastfeed your baby successfully.

Breastfeeding changes day by day, and there's no right and wrong way to do it that matches every situation. Here we give the basic information about how it works, and what your expectations might be – not a blueprint for you to follow.

THE FIRST FEED

Unless you or your baby need immediate and urgent medical attention, you can feed your baby immediately after the birth. It doesn't matter if you have had a caesarean section (see page 38); if your baby has been born with the help of forceps or a ventouse; if you have had pain relief; or if you have had a long or even very quick labour. You can hold your baby close and offer her the chance to come to your breast and feed.

Not all newborn babies seem very keen on actually feeding – they may be affected by the birth, or the pain relief you have had, and be sleepy, or not show much interest in the breast. But in most maternity units today, the midwife who has helped you give birth will be happy to help you get into a comfortable position so that your baby can take the chance to start getting to know you – your smell, your face, your voice – and enjoy the warm, secure feeling of being close to your breast.

Warning!

Even at this early stage, you may need to be very careful that your baby is positioned in a way that doesn't damage your nipples. See pages 32–35.

THE ROOTING REFLEX

Alert babies will show the 'rooting' reflex. This means that your baby seems to look for the breast by turning her head and opening her mouth and making sucking movements – really 'looking for' the breast. She is also able to suck and swallow – both reflexes present at birth – so she is truly geared up for feeding.

If you put her to the breast, your baby's sucking will also stimulate the release of oxytocin – the hormone that causes contractions. This helps your uterus expel the placenta.

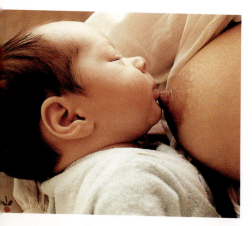
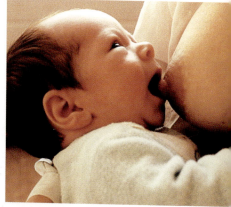

HOW YOU GET READY TO BREASTFEED

When your baby first comes to the breast, she is rewarded with colostrum, which is in your breasts at the time of the birth. Her sucking also stimulates the breasts to produce milk (see pages 26–29). As soon as the placenta is delivered, your body responds by producing prolactin – the milk-making hormone – and over the following few days the colostrum will gradually be replaced with milk.

Use this time to say 'hello' to your baby, and to enjoy the peace and the sense of joy you get at greeting your new son or daughter. Just be patient – give your baby time to decide if she wants to feed or not, and don't worry if she doesn't seem to 'do' much. There's no rush.

WHAT IS COLOSTRUM?

Your breasts produce colostrum, a highly valuable fluid, rich in antibodies, to meet the needs of your very new baby. It has laxative properties, and helps your baby get rid of the meconium in her bowel. It prepares her digestive tract for breast milk, and the antibodies it contains give her a unique protection against the risks of her new environment – the outside world. The colour of colostrum varies. It may be thick and creamy looking, or thinner and pale yellow like straw, transparent or opaque. It's been called 'liquid gold'.

There is not a huge amount of colostrum – new babies don't normally need or want a lot of fluids. Even if you don't intend to breastfeed, it is worth giving your baby colostrum.

2

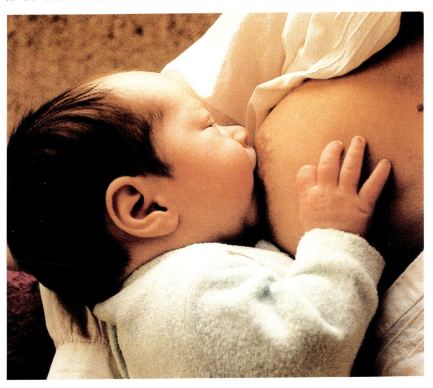

MAKING BREAST MILK

Y ou make milk for your baby whether or not you intend to breastfeed. The 'breast-milk production line' gets under way, and by day two, three or four (sometimes more) after the birth, the colostrum in your breasts is replaced with milk. This happens under the influence of the milk-making hormone, prolactin. If your baby is pre-term, you will still make milk within a few days of birth: the breasts are capable of making milk after about six months of pregnancy

2

LET DOWN

Breast milk is made in the breasts and stored in little pockets called alveoli. The alveoli lead to ducts, down which the milk travels, and as the baby suckles it appears through tiny holes in the end of the nipple. There are small 'reservoirs' just behind the nipple, where milk pools in instant readiness for the baby, any place, any time.

However, to feed effectively, the baby needs to make sure that the milk stored in the breast comes down the ducts, too. This happens with the let down reflex, known simply as 'let down', when the milk is literally let down from the alveoli. It's also called the milk ejection reflex.

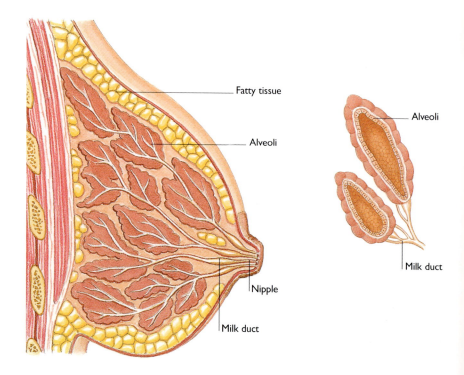

Fatty tissue

Alveoli

Alveoli

Milk duct

Nipple

Milk duct

2

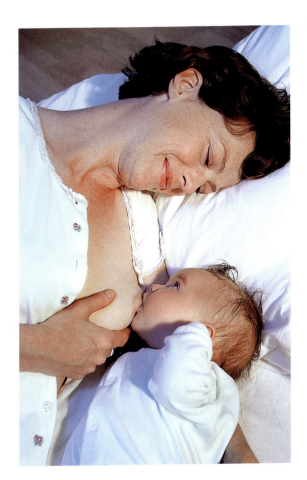

IS LET DOWN PAINFUL?

No. Some women may feel a slight, non-painful tingling in their breasts or a feeling like a warmth or a rush of milk, and some feel nothing.

In the very early days, there may be after-pains in the uterus, since breastfeeding encourages it to contract. But this is natural, and it is another way that breastfeeding can help you.

If there is any pain, it is not usually anything more than brief and fleeting. If it's more than this, it is safe for you to take some paracetamol.

HOW LET DOWN WORKS

When your baby comes to the breast, if she's positioned in the correct way (see pages 32–35), the action of her jaws, tongue and mouth stimulates nerve endings in the nipple. These transmit a message to the pituitary gland at the base of the brain to secrete the hormone oxytocin, which travels via the blood stream to the breasts.

Oxytocin is the hormone that causes the uterus to contract and, ultimately, to help push your baby out during labour and birth. It functions in a similar way during breastfeeding – but this time, the oxytocin works directly on the tiny muscle cells of the alveoli.

The muscle cells contract, and this literally pushes the milk out, and down into the ducts. When let down is working very well, it happens pretty soon after the baby starts to suckle and can sometimes be quite forceful, causing the milk to shoot out in a stream or in spurts.

WILL I HAVE ENOUGH MILK?

The very act of feeding makes more milk for your baby. Removing milk from your breasts by feeding your baby 'tells' your body to make more to replace it. In fact, leaving milk in the breasts without removing it reduces the supply. This is because milk itself contains a hormone that puts a brake on production and that's why, contrary to expectations, leaving long gaps between feeds does not give your breasts time to fill up. In fact, it reduces the milk supply, since you're sending the wrong messages to your body – in effect, you're saying 'make less', not more. In the short term, your breasts will feel fuller; in the longer term, it means a reduced supply.

2

LET YOUR BABY SET THE PACE

Leaving your baby to suckle when she wants to, rather than timing her feeds by the clock will:

■ ensure that your body understands more milk is needed.

■ keep you comfortable, so you don't allow milk to build up.

■ ensure that your baby gets the hind milk she needs – taking her off before she is ready may prevent this and also prevent you making enough milk.

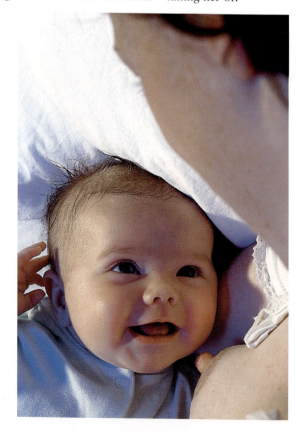

Remember, you will naturally make milk for your baby, but your body knows to continue making it only if you 'tell' it to do so by feeding your baby, or by expressing your milk (see pages 58–59).

By sucking effectively (see pages 32–35), the baby also plays an important part. The let down reflex is stimulated and the reservoirs inside the breast are 'milked' by her tongue and jaw.

You and your baby are a partnership, learning together to make sure your body works well for both of you.

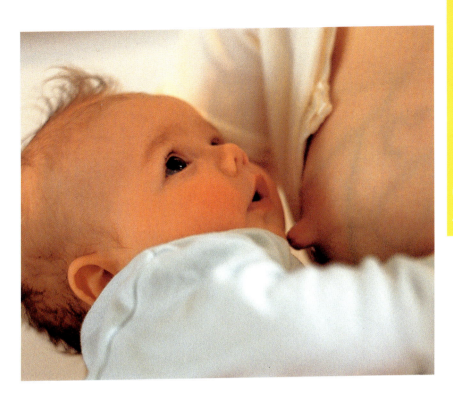

FORE MILK AND HIND MILK

The milk that's available at the start of the feed, and is already in the reservoirs and the ducts in your breasts, has a high proportion of water in it. The milk in the storage cells is fattier. This is not because the breasts make two different sorts of milk. It's all the same milk, but the fattier constituents of the milk tend to stick to the alveoli and need the stimulus of the let down to be pushed out.

You don't need to be concerned that your baby won't get her milk in the right proportions. Just let her stay on the breast for as long as she wants to, and feed her when she seems to 'ask' for it, and she will sort out the balance herself. However, if you deliberately take her off the breast after an arbitrary time limit, you may end up limiting the amount of hind milk she gets. This is one of the reasons why babies on a strict schedule, who are only 'allowed' to feed for a certain time, may not thrive. They don't get the calorie-rich hind milk they need to grow.

THE ULTIMATE CONVENIENCE FOOD!

The more you feed, the more milk you make. This response means that mothers who have twins make twice as much milk (see pages 96–97) because they are feeding twice as much, and why mothers of babies who aren't feeding well, or at all, may need to express milk to make sure the 'message' to keep producing gets to their breasts.

FIRST DAYS

The normal way to care for your new baby – the way humans have done it for thousands of generations – is to stay close to her, and to give her plenty of opportunities to come to your breast and to get to know you. The more usual way after a hospital birth is for you to be in bed, and for your baby to be away from you in a plastic crib, tucked up not against your body but under a sheet and a blanket.

Many babies sleep for long periods after the birth. This is more likely to happen if you have had certain forms of pain relief such as diamorphine. The difficulty here is that sleeping for a long time delays effective breastfeeding, and this can mean that establishing it is more of a challenge.

Whether your baby is sleepy or not, keep her close to you, tucked up with you in bed or sitting in your chair. She won't need a lot of wrapping or clothing, but can be kept warm next to your skin as you hold and cuddle her, while you start to get to know each other.

2

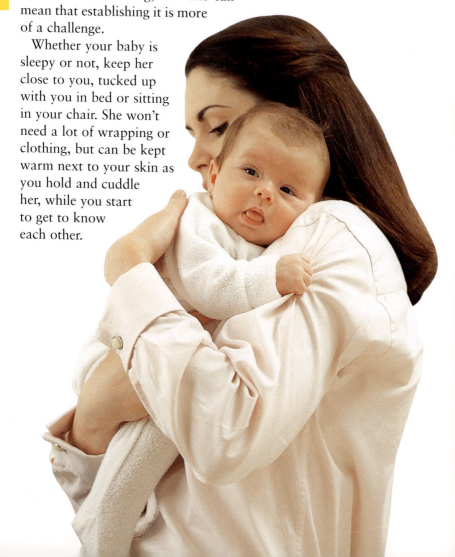

LEARNING TO BREASTFEED

Unless you are very sure of yourself, ask someone to help you get your baby comfortably positioned at the breast. You may need some assistance to sit up, or lie comfortably, especially if you have had stitches or a caesarean section. For details of exactly how your baby takes the breast and feeds happily and effectively, see pages 32-35.

Don't be worried if everything feels awkward at first. You will get better and better – and breastfeeding is usually very frequent, especially in the first days, so you and your baby will become more skilled, hour by hour. There is no desperate rush for everything to be perfect – if you don't get it right straightaway, you don't need to feel anxious.

YOUR MILK COMES IN

At any time between day two and day four, sometimes later, your milk comes in. This is the surge of production that means your breasts have started making milk, and because there is more milk, in terms of volume, than colostrum, you may feel your breasts are a lot fuller than before. In fact, it's not just milk that fills them. A great increase in blood supply and fluid also 'swells' the breasts in the days just after the birth.

If your baby is feeding a lot, and sucking and swallowing effectively, you may not notice this change as much more than 'feeling fuller', but a few women who produce a lot of milk, or whose babies are not yet feeding often, may experience engorgement. This is an uncomfortable, swollen feeling that leads to hard, tender breasts and possible difficulties for the baby with taking the breast, since it is so large and hard.

Engorgement almost always passes as your baby starts to feed more and takes off the 'extra' milk. If you need more help, see pages 70–71.

YOUR BABY CHANGES, TOO

It's very common for a sleepy baby to perk up after the first couple of days, and be more alert than before – and more hungry. You will see how your milk, and her intake change, by the changes that occur in her stools.

As her bowels clear, and she goes on to digest your milk and metabolize it, she will go from passing black to brown to green to yellow stools. In fact, bright yellow, soft stools are sometimes known as 'breast-milk stools'.

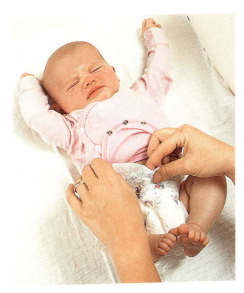

GETTING IT RIGHT

You've got the milk, your baby wants it – getting those two elements to work together shouldn't be too hard, yet some of the most common problems experienced by breastfeeding mothers are concerned with just that.

LATCHING ON

Latching on – getting your baby to take the breast effectively and happily without a fuss or a struggle – is essential to successful breastfeeding. 'My baby wouldn't latch on', or 'My nipples were so sore', or 'She wouldn't stay latched on' are common reasons why mothers report that breastfeeding was difficult – so difficult for some that they made the switch to the bottle.

Later, as your baby grows, you'll be able to breastfeed without thinking twice about positioning. But while you and your baby are learning, you may need to think carefully about it. Here's how to ensure your baby latches on in a way that's pain-free for you, and which brings her the contentment of a satisfying feed.

■ Make sure you are sitting comfortably, with your shoulders relaxed, a cold drink at hand. It helps to wear light, easy-to-manage clothing, so you aren't coping with layers of sweaters or tight tops.

■ Hold your baby chest-to-chest with you, with her lying across your body. If it helps to have a pillow on your lap while you are learning, then have one. Experiment with and without.

■ Your baby shouldn't have to turn or lift her head to feed. When her mouth is closed, her nose should be at the same level as your nipple. This is not the case if her mouth is already open – as it often will be if she is keen on feeding.

■ When your baby's mouth is wide open, bring her on to your breast, aiming the nipple toward the upper part of her mouth.

If she is on correctly, it won't hurt you, although some women do experience some pain even with a good latch (see pages 68–69), and she will be able to use her tongue and her jaw to remove the milk. Her chin will be touching the lower half of your breast and her nose will be against the upper half.

REMEMBER!

Chest to chest, and baby to breast. Don't try to chase your baby's mouth with your nipple, or post it into her half-open mouth. You may manage to get it in, but you'll be sore and your baby may not be able to suck effectively.

Latching on incorrectly

Latching on correctly

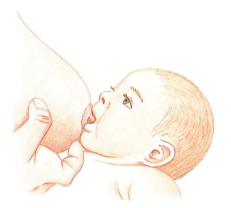

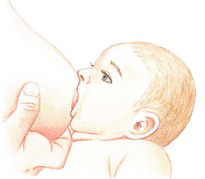

DON'T

■ Try to feed your baby if she is crying or screaming – babies who are adept at breastfeeding can change the position of the tongue as they come on to the breast, but babies who are still learning cannot latch on if they are crying because the tongue is too far back in the mouth. If she is crying, your baby needs comforting first.

■ Try to pull your baby's chin down to get a better latch – the only effective way is for her to do it herself.

■ Be worried if you and your baby have to try again and again.

■ Be anxious about your baby's nose being buried in your breast (that's what it looks like, sometimes). Her nostrils are flared and her nose is snub, so breathing is easy at the breast.

■ Place your fingers near the nipple, or anywhere they could interfere with your baby getting a good mouthful.

■ Press your fingers into your breasts – it could distort the shape of your nipple in your baby's mouth.

ALWAYS

■ Remove your baby if is she is not latched on correctly and try again.

■ Consciously relax yourself so that you're not feeding with hunched shoulders or tension in your arms.

■ Ask someone who knows what to look for to check that your baby is properly latched on if you are not sure about it.

2

IS SHE ON RIGHT?

Check whether your baby is latched on correctly by watching her suck, as well as by gauging your own comfort. She will probably start to suck quickly, and then settle into a slower sucking and swallowing pattern which involves her whole jaw. It needs to, since she's got a large mouthful of breast in there!

In fact, your nipple is right at the back of her mouth; when it isn't, it can cause you a lot of pain, since the nipple tip then rubs against the baby's hard palate. You can see the jaw muscles working at the side of her face. Every so often she may start to suck more quickly again, and then settle down once more. For information on helping a baby who refuses to feed, see pages 64–67.

OTHER HELPFUL TIPS

■ Some babies hate to be wrapped when feeding. Leave their arms free.

■ Others are distracted by their own waving arms, and their hands get in the way. You may need to use a sheet or a wrap while your baby is learning if she is like this.

■ If you have large breasts, or soft breasts, it may be more comfortable for you to support the breast from underneath with your hand.

■ If you are engorged (see page 31), you may need to soften your breasts by gently expressing some milk (see pages 58–59); this will help your baby to latch on more easily.

■ Make sure clothing – yours or your baby's – is not hindering you; sometimes folds of cloth bunch up and get in the way.

GOOD POSITIONING

When your baby is in the right position it will help:

■ to avoid sore and cracked nipples

■ to ensure good breastfeeding, with stimulation of the let down reflex, efficient removal of milk and, therefore, stimulation of a good supply, and the avoidance of blocked ducts and mastitis (see pages 68–71)

■ to ensure a happy baby, who feels comfortable and confident and keen on feeding from the breast

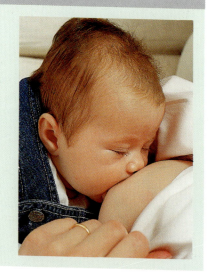

SLEEPING

In the early days and weeks, your baby will probably sleep several times during the day and night, and there will be at least a short sleep between, and sometimes during, breastfeeds.

After the first week or two, she may have a longer uninterrupted sleep at night, but night feeds are not only normal they are essential for a very young baby. So you must expect to feed your baby two or three times in the time you are in bed yourself – sleeping in the same bed with your baby, or in the same room, makes night feeds easier.

Sometimes you will think your baby has fallen asleep on the breast. She comes off, looks fast asleep and appears to want to stay that way. But if, after just a minute or two, she comes round and wants some more time on the breast, that's fine!

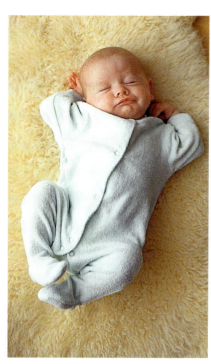

2

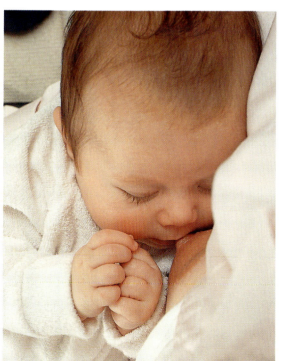

LONG FEEDS

Feeds are not normal when the baby seems to take more than, say, 40 minutes to be anything like satisfied, and then wants to feed again shortly afterwards, without ever seeming to be truly content.

The occasional long feed like this is fine – it's when it's a consistent pattern that it gives cause for concern. Feeds that take such a long time may be a sign that you need help with your breastfeeding (see pages 62–63).

BABIES IN SPECIAL CARE

2

About one in every seven babies spends some time in special care, and while in most cases the stay is brief, it still means an interruption to the usual course of events – when you can feed your baby when she seems to want it. If your baby is in special care, discuss her feeding and care with the staff, and let them know you aim to breastfeed.

If you can't feed your baby directly from the breast, you need to express. A midwife will show you what to do. At first, you can express colostrum, probably by hand and into a little cup because of the small volume. Later, if you prefer, you can use a pump. Your baby can take your milk by tube, in a syringe, by sipping or lapping from a cup, or by bottle and teat.

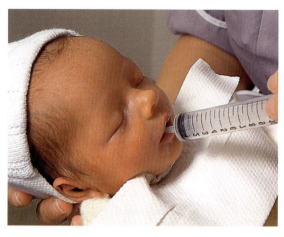

No one is sure if the so-called 'nipple–teat confusion' actually exists, since some babies develop both sucking skills without a problem. However, the bottle makes it easier to get larger volumes into the baby, and this may disturb the way she learns about feeding – she ends up expecting more every time.

Keeping breastfeeding going when your baby isn't able to feed often, or at all, means regular expressing. You should aim to express several times a day – between six and eight times, including once at night.

CAESAREAN SECTION

Having had a caesarean section doesn't have to make a serious difference to your breastfeeding. It used to be thought that a general anaesthetic delayed the milk coming in, but this doesn't seem to be the case today. In any event, you are much more likely to have had an epidural than a general anaesthetic.

The main challenge to happy breastfeeding after a caesarean is getting comfortable. You'll have stitches and a sore tummy, perhaps discomfort with wind, and you will probably feel more 'wiped out' than after a vaginal birth. So you'll need more help in getting your baby latched on correctly and finding a position in which you feel relaxed. But these are all features of the early days – they soon pass as you become pain-free and more confident.

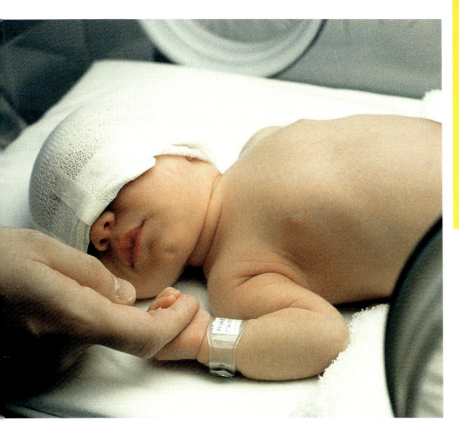

YOUR BABY IN SPECIAL CARE NEEDS YOUR MILK

■ Feeding her is the unique thing you can do for her, in the middle of what might be a medical or nursing situation where other people, even machines, are playing a central role.

■ Breast milk is a powerful weapon against infection – and tiny, vulnerable babies are even more at risk than healthy ones.

■ In particular, necrotizing enterocolitis, a disease of the gut which can be especially dangerous to small, sick babies, has been shown to be far more common in those who receive no breast milk.

In some situations, the paediatrician looking after your baby may want to ensure that she gets more than just your milk, and you may be advised that, temporarily, formula should be added to your baby's diet. But this does not mean you can't breastfeed fully later on.

There is more information about expressing milk, and about caring for your pre-term baby in hospital and at home on pages 58–59 and 98–99.

CONFIDENCE CHECKLIST

How do you know breastfeeding's going well with your new baby? Check these points after the first few days – you should be able to answer 'yes' to every question.

■ Is my baby alert and keen to feed at least six to eight times a day?

■ Is she producing several wet nappies a day?

■ Are her stools changing day by day? Have they become soft and yellow by days five to seven or sooner?

■ Does she come off the breast by herself and look contented?

■ Is my baby waking at least twice at night? (So that even at night she doesn't regularly go longer than three to four hours without a feed.)

■ Are my nipples pain-free and not cracked? From day one, your nipples should not be sore without you asking someone to check your positioning (see pages 66–67).

■ Do my breasts show no signs of severe hardness or engorgement? (A feeling of fullness, especially just before you feed your baby, is normal.)

2

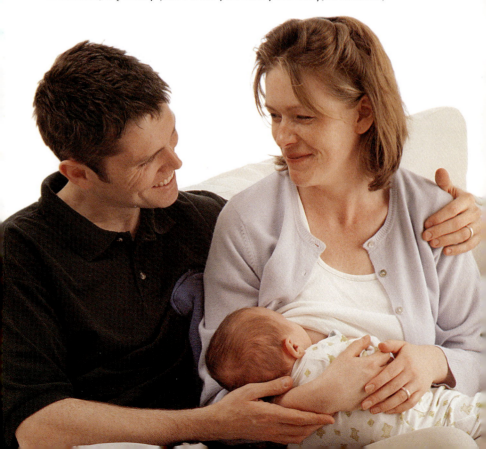

EVERYDAY BREASTFEEDING

The best and happiest sort of breastfeeding takes place without your worrying about whether you're doing it right, without anxiety about the baby, and under as little pressure and stress as possible.

Once you and your baby have learned this new skill together, breastfeeding should be a relaxed, normal and natural part of caring for your baby. It should be something you both enjoy and should fit in well with all the other things you might want and need to do.

Here we see whether some aspects of your life need adjustment; whether you need to do anything special to ensure breastfeeding success; and how other members of the family may react to your breastfeeding. We also consider how your baby's crying and pattern of sleeping and waking affect breastfeeding.

AFTER THE EARLY DAYS

We've seen on pages 26–29 how the breast milk 'production line' needs to be 'told' to continue – and how the more you feed, the more milk you make. It's very important to keep that in mind as the weeks go by.

Trying to mix bottles, or formula, with breastfeeding is not usually an ideal way to ensure successful breastfeeding, although it can be done when your baby is older (see pages 86–87). Give yourself, your baby, and your body, a chance to get breastfeeding established by sticking to breastfeeding alone at first.

Apart from the known advantages of breastfeeding without giving anything else until the baby is old enough for solid food (see pages 80–81), giving bottles undermines your breastfeeding and reduces your chances of continuing. One British study revealed that mothers who introduced bottles while in hospital were three times more likely to be bottle feeding entirely by the time their babies were two weeks old than mothers who only breastfed in hospital. Experts observe that once a mother starts giving bottles in addition to a breastfeed, or instead of a breastfeed, this often leads to her giving up breastfeeding altogether.

3

WHY IS THIS SO?

■ Giving formula milk fills up the baby's tummy and reduces his hunger, making him less likely to wake and need another breast feed – so the stimulation of the breast is reduced, and without this stimulation the supply of milk is reduced.

■ The teat provokes a different sucking action from the baby, and the milk comes out of the bottle in a different way. For a baby whose experience at the breast has not been very good, this may mean that he prefers the bottle. Some people think this is 'nipple–teat confusion' – others say that the baby is making a choice

■ Your own reactions to the situation also play a part. Giving bottles can mean that you lose confidence in breastfeeding, especially if your baby seems more settled and sleepy after he has had a bottle feed.

EXPRESSING

You can express breast milk at any time, and it's essential to do so if your baby is unable to come to the breast or has severe sucking difficulties.

Expressing will help to establish a good supply of milk. But there is no special virtue in expressing – and if you are keen to build up your milk supply, your baby's sucking is the best way to stimulate it.

ESTABLISHING BREASTFEEDING

You can help breastfeeding to become established by:

■ feeding your baby whenever you want to, or whenever he seems to want to come to the breast.

■ keeping your baby close to you so that you can respond to his cues.

■ avoiding the use of formula milk, water, juice or anything other than breast milk.

■ avoiding the use of dummies (pacifiers) until at least a few weeks have passed. With some babies, dummies can satisfy their sucking needs and therefore reduce the time they spend on the breast – leading to a lessening of the milk supply.

■ feeding at night. Sleeping with your baby is fine, as long as you don't smoke; as long as neither you nor your partner are drunk or drugged; and as long as your baby doesn't get too hot.

3

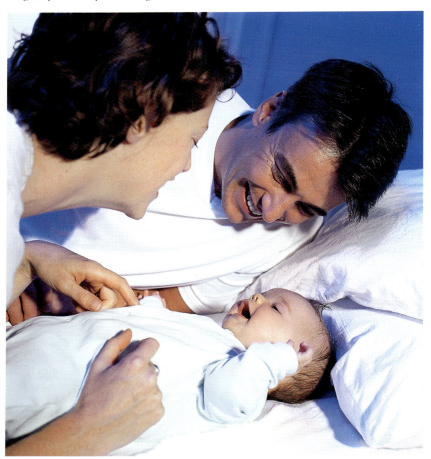

CHANGES TO EXPECT

Breastfeeding is an evolving process. It changes over weeks, months and years if you continue with it. Just as your relationship with your baby develops, your breastfeeding responds to his changing needs.

CHANGES TO YOUR BREASTS

■ At first, your breasts will feel fuller than they did before the birth (see page 31), but after a day or so they will become softer. Why?

The first surge of milk, blood and fluid to the breasts makes them fuller; then, when the baby feeds more frequently, the milk is removed.

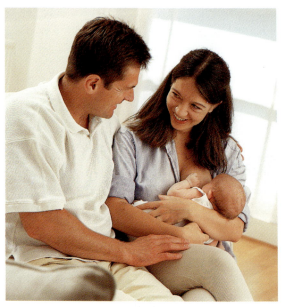

■ For a few weeks or more they may feel full before a feed and noticeably softer afterwards. Why?

Initially, if you feed your baby unrestrictedly, your body tends to make 'extra' milk, producing milk between feeds as well as during the feeds. This means you store the milk, and when the baby feeds much of the milk is removed (although you can never truly empty the breasts).

■ After a few weeks – the length of time varies enormously from woman to woman, and anywhere between 2 and 12 weeks or more is normal – your breasts will seem softer most of the time. Why?

This happens when breastfeeding is established because much of the milk is made when the baby feeds, and there is less actual production between feeds. If you didn't know that this was normal, you might even think 'Where's my milk?' (see pages 84–85).

■ If you stop breastfeeding after a while, your breasts seem even softer and smaller than they were pre-pregnancy. Why?

Because, by now, much of the fat that gives the breasts their shape when they're not actually lactating has been replaced with milk production and storage tissue – and it takes time for the fat to be laid down again.

CHANGES IN YOUR MILK

Your milk is not identical at every feed and at all times of the day. Studies have shown that the fat content, for instance, differs between mothers and between feeds, and during feeds. More frequent feeding increases the fat content of the milk.

Protein levels of breast milk fall throughout the first year, regardless of what the mother herself eats. Nature has 'designed' the milk this way, since it meets the physiological way your baby is 'designed' to grow.

THE ROLE OF PROLACTIN

When breastfeeding is getting under way, the hormone prolactin is very important in the production of milk. But prolactin levels actually fall throughout the first months after the birth, and by the time your baby is six months old, they're back to normal, non-lactating levels.

Yet you are capable of producing a lot of milk at this time. The process is not yet fully understood, but it appears that established milk production depends on the removal of milk and the act of feeding, and it has less and less to do with prolactin.

This explains why women can bring back their milk after a period of non-breastfeeding – as long as the baby cooperates by coming to the breast frequently. There may be no prolactin in the mother's circulation at all, but the very act of stimulating the breasts by suckling is sufficient (see pages 84–85).

3

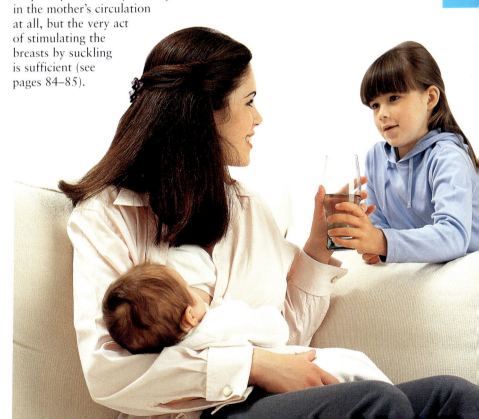

CARING FOR YOURSELF

The good news is that you really don't have to be worried about your food and drink intake while you are breastfeeding.

Women all over the world on many different diets breastfeed, making good-quality milk for their babies no matter what they eat and drink. However, research has shown that the quality and quantity of breast milk may falter when mothers are on extremely low-calorie diets, so it is not a good idea to restrict calories too much when you're breastfeeding, for your own sake, as well as your baby's. But in normal circumstances, production of breast milk depends on your baby feeding frequently enough to stimulate your body to make the milk.

I'M MORE HUNGRY WHEN I BREASTFEED...

That's normal! Breastfeeding does use up energy stores, and you may often feel that you need to eat something to prevent yourself from being hungry – just eat what you feel you need.

It's impossible to say how many 'extra' calories you need when you breastfeed. It's not correct to work out the calorific value of a day's worth of breast milk and then equate that with the amount of calories a mother needs to make it. For one thing, she's laid down extra fat in pregnancy to compensate, and for another, the body seems to be very efficient at using calories during this time – it gives out more than it needs to take in.

3

EAT WHAT YOU LIKE

The advice to avoid foods such as pâtés, unpasteurized cheeses and milk while you are pregnant (because of the small risk of listeria) does not apply while you are breastfeeding. The bacterium in the cheese does not reach the breast milk.

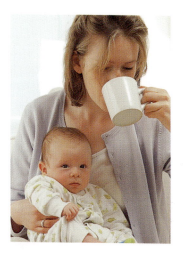

...AND I'M THIRSTIER

Normal, too! It is extremely common to have a raging thirst actually during a feed, so it's useful to have a drink of something cold (for safety's sake) at your side while you are feeding. Most mothers find this thirst tends to disappear as time goes on.

EATING SPECIAL FOODS

No food has been shown to have any special 'milk-making' property, although many cultures throughout the world have foods that are reputed to be good for the milk. Just eat what you like.

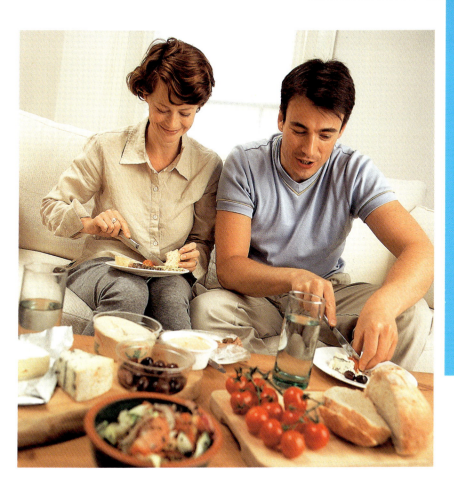

3

AVOIDING CERTAIN FOODS

It is not usually necessary to avoid any foods, although mothers with colicky babies (see pages 54–55) may want to try adjusting their diets to see if it makes a difference. It does appear that some constituents of foods affect the breast milk – how, we don't really know.

There has been some research on dairy products, and removing these from the mother's diet has been shown to help with babies suffering from colic. If you think there may be some connection between what you eat and symptoms in your baby, get professional support and advice on altering your diet.

ALCOHOL

Alcohol does reach the breast milk, but no research has shown any long-term harm to babies who have been fed by mothers who drink moderately.

If you feel concerned about alcohol and your breast milk, the cautious advice would be to feed your baby before you have a drink. When you are no longer affected by alcohol, it's also gone from your milk.

YOUR FEELINGS

L earning how to feed, and getting the positioning right, becoming more familiar with your baby and his needs, and understanding how you make milk, are all important to happy breastfeeding – but the way you feel about it, and the support of other people, also play a part in successful breastfeeding.

If you find breastfeeding difficult, you may feel very low, and possibly guilty. You could even feel a failure as a mother and a woman. This isn't rational, of course – breastfeeding problems are not your fault, and most occur because of lack of good information or support, or problems with the baby being ill or having sucking difficulties. You may even decide you're selfish, wanting to do something that doesn't keep your baby satisfied or happy, or which seems to present him with a challenge he can't meet.

IF YOU FEEL LIKE GIVING UP

3

Try to get support from people who will help you decide what is right for you, without pushing you one way or the other. If it is important for you to breastfeed, then stopping is a big decision and not to be taken lightly. See pages 108–110 for a discussion about stopping.

In reality, there's not a lot of support for breastfeeding, despite the fact that almost everyone accepts that 'breast is best'. Bottle feeding is now so common, and is regarded as being so normal, that you may find people wonder why on earth you are 'bothering', especially if you strike problems.

Finding friends who have breastfed, and other mothers who are doing it now, can really help you (see pages 76–78).

IT'S NOT ALL BAD

In fact, breastfeeding usually isn't bad at all, even if you do experience problems. It helps you to feel close to your baby and good about yourself as a mother. You can feel proud of doing this for your baby, and later on look back on the experience as a positive, meaningful one.

HOW DOES BREASTFEEDING AFFECT YOUR SEX LIFE?

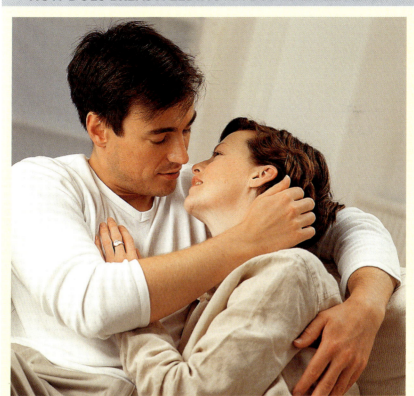

3

Breastfeeding can be a warm, loving, relaxing and sensual experience. Very occasionally, women report that it engenders true sexual arousal. That's fine – it's all part of the wonderful diversity of human experience.

There's great variation in the possible sexual effects of breastfeeding. Does it make you feel more or less like having sex with your partner? Some women say they feel less like it, and their desire comes back when they stop. According to other women, their sexual feelings are entirely unaffected. In any event, it is difficult to link this with breastfeeding itself, since caring for a new baby and the change in lifestyle and outlook this brings can also affect your sexual feelings.

Tiredness, too, is an issue. There is research to indicate that women who breastfeed resume sexual relations sooner than women who bottle feed – but this may mean nothing more than that women who are comfortable with their bodies and their sexuality may be more likely to breastfeed than bottle feed.

The hormonal effects of breastfeeding are hard to pin down. Some women say they notice their natural vaginal lubrication is affected and they need to use a product such as KY jelly or Astroglide to help. It might be, however, that lack of lubrication is due to post-childbirth effects, or lack of sexual interest, or simply to the natural bodily changes that take place as we get older.

EFFECTS ON THE FAMILY

Having a new baby means that everyone has to make changes. Some mothers become anxious that breastfeeding could make their partners feel jealous, for two reasons. First, fathers may feel excluded from the relationship and worried that they may not get close to their baby or 'bond' with him; and second, they may feel that the baby has 'taken over' their partner's breasts.

If you think either of these could be an issue with your partner, talk about it, perhaps during pregnancy.

Many men like the idea of their baby getting such a good start in life, and are truly unconcerned about being excluded. They also recognize that bonding is a gradual process, which takes place in many ways and does not depend on being able to offer a feed. Being jealous of the baby's 'use' of their partner's breasts is not an issue – or if it is, it's one they can cope with very well.

3

A FATHER'S BOND WITH HIS BABY

Exclusive breastfeeding lasts only four to six months. Even in that time there are many things a man can do to nurture his relationship with his baby – indeed, he can do everything a mother can except feed. A father can develop his own relationship with his baby, parallel to the mother's relationship.

In addition, it is very important for a father to offer his loving support and encouragement to the breastfeeding mother and baby. Research shows that a father's positive feelings about breastfeeding are crucial in determining whether the mother chooses to breastfeed in the first place, and then chooses to continue with it.

For a while, the new baby's needs come first in most families, and everyone else has to take second place. But they soon learn to understand that although breastfeeding can be very time-consuming initially, this period doesn't last long.

DEPRESSION AFTER CHILDBIRTH

Post-natal depression affects 12 to 15 per cent of new mothers and probably a smaller, but unknown, proportion of new fathers as well.

It is very common to feel overwhelmed by new parenthood from time to time and to have fleeting feelings that you are a bad parent. However, if these feelings last and you can't overcome them, they may be a sign of depression.

If either you or your partner suspect that you are suffering from depression, seek help from your family doctor or your health visitor.

'MY TODDLER IS SO JEALOUS OF THE NEW BABY – MAYBE I SHOULD BOTTLE FEED'

One of the nice things about breastfeeding is that it leaves you with a spare arm, with which you can cuddle the toddler, hold a book to share, and even build a brick tower or a Lego house. Encourage your toddler to see feed times not as a threat, but as times when you can sit down and pay attention to him as well. You also need to build in some time during the day or the evening when you can give your toddler one-to-one attention – perhaps when the baby is in someone else's arms or asleep. A few minutes will be fine, as long as it is often enough – at least once every day.

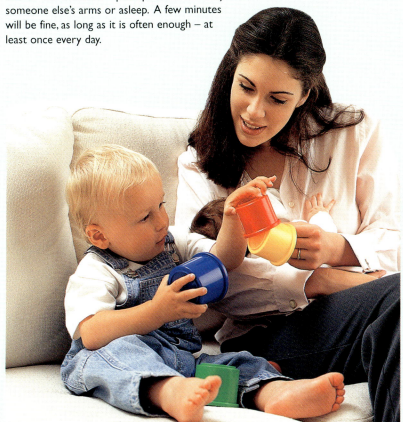

3

'MY TODDLER WANTS TO FEED, TOO – SHALL I LET HIM?'

He's probably just curious. Give him a turn! He's unlikely to want to take it up again and may not have the right technique any more. For information on feeding a baby and a toddler – known as tandem feeding – see pages **88–89** and **107**.

HOW OTHER PEOPLE FEEL

People have strong feelings about breastfeeding an infant – and they don't always keep their criticisms to themselves.

For some, breastfeeding may never seem like a healthy option. If they don't know the facts about its benefits, they may assume there's something 'germy' about a baby sucking on flesh, taking in fluid the mother makes in her own body. They may even that feel that breast milk is a body fluid like mucus, urine or saliva – something not quite nice.

THE SEXUAL ASPECT

Women's breasts are a source of sexual pleasure to men, and to women themselves. This sexual aspect is sometimes exploited in newspapers and in advertisements. Breasts are sexually alluring – and some people feel uncomfortable at the sight, or even the thought, that they may have a nurturing function as well.

The upshot of this is that breastfeeding mothers may be asked, or expected, to feed their babies in private. To feed where other people can see what you're doing is regarded as exhibitionist, embarrassing and rude.

SO WHAT SHOULD MOTHERS DO?

It's really your choice whether you go along with this view and decide to feed in private, where no one can be embarrassed, critical or confused. But the counter-argument is a strong one.

To breastfeed is to do nothing more than to give your baby sustenance and comfort – and if people have a problem with that then, of course, they can go somewhere else, or simply not look.

Even in societies where women are expected to dress 'modestly' and to keep flesh under cover, breastfeeding is accepted as a natural and necessary thing, and no one would expect a mother to feel awkward about it. 'Public' breastfeeding is an everyday sight.

There's also a practical argument. Just where can you feed your baby if you can't feed in front of anyone who may be disturbed by it?

Young babies may need feeding at any time, and it may not be easy to find somewhere clean and comfortable to sit and do it. The ladies' lavatory in a public building is not a pleasant place to feed, and if you have shopping and other children with you, it is not at all convenient.

If you're in someone's house, you may be asked to go to another room – it means you're not part of the company while you are feeding, but it is polite to respect people's wishes when you are in their home.

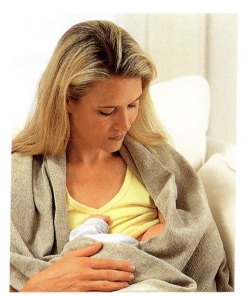

DON'T HIDE AWAY!

The more women who feel relaxed and confident about feeding where they happen to be, the better it is for every mother who wants to breastfeed her baby.

Practise your breastfeeding in front of a mirror, so you know that you can do it without looking hampered by clothing. It's very much easier to breastfeed if you have a top you can lift up from the waist, rather than a dress that fastens down the back.

If you suspect that there are members of your family who are embarrassed by your breastfeeding, consider talking to them about it, and explaining some of the benefits to your baby. Don't feel obliged to make a point by feeding in front of them if you think it's too big a step for you to take. But give it some thought, and perhaps ask for your partner's support.

3

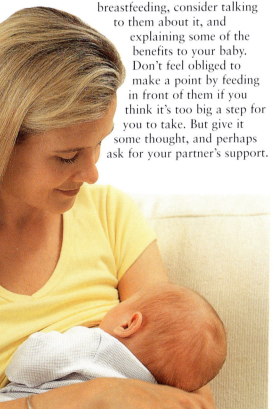

WHY DOES MY BABY CRY?

Some babies cry a great deal and take time to be calmed and soothed, and then they may not stay calm for long. If you have a baby like this, you may feel his distress is connected with breastfeeding – and it is possible that fixing the breastfeeding will indeed help your baby to become happier.

Regular bouts of inconsolable crying, especially prolonged bouts in the early evening, are also a characteristic of colic. Some experts feel that the crying is a sign of wind in the tummy, causing a feeling of fullness and pain. Although it is wearing and upsetting for you, both crying and colic tend to get better by themselves by the time the baby is about three months old. In the meantime, ask your doctor or chemist to recommend some anti-colic medication for your baby.

CAN BABIES PICK UP TENSION?

There is some evidence to suggest that this is so. One study found that colic was far more prevalent in babies whose parents had suffered stress during pregnancy and who experienced negative feelings about the birth.

The researchers recommended more support for parents, to increase their confidence in their ability to care for their babies.

Family therapists giving counselling to parents of crying babies report that as the parents' confidence increases and their anxiety reduces, the babies' distressed behaviour also changes.

IS IT SOMETHING IN THE MILK?

Dairy products in the mother's diet may produce symptoms in her baby, and a few studies implicate tea, coffee and cola in the babies' periodic fussiness and general restlessness

If your baby's crying seems to be linked to something you're eating, try cutting out the offending food for a few days to see if there's any improvement.

But make quite sure that you don't go short of vital foods yourself.

OSTEOPATHY

Babies who cry a lot and are difficult to console are sometimes helped by osteopathy.

It appears that miserable babies may be uncomfortable and even in pain because their bones (especially of the neck, back or skull) have been affected by the birth.

Gentle, skilled and knowledgeable touching and maybe manipulation can put things right for these babies, and they become more settled.

If you think your baby might be helped by this, see a qualified osteopath with experience in treating babies and small children. Your health visitor may know of local therapists, or you can ask other parents for their recommendation.

CRYING CHECKLIST

If your baby is crying and you can't seem to soothe him, go through this checklist – it may help you to find out what is wrong with him.

■ Is he hungry? This is the most common reason for crying. Let your baby decide when to come off the first breast if you're breastfeeding. Then offer the other breast.

■ Is he thirsty? Offer the breast – the perfect food and drink. Is he getting a satisfying feed? Check your baby's position on the breast to make sure he's stimulating the let down reflex which brings him the calorie-rich hind milk.

■ Does he need 'winding'? Sit your baby in an upright position and gently rub his back.

■ Is he too hot or too cold? Check his chest; it should feel comfortably warm, not hot and clammy or cold.

■ Is he tired, yet unable to sleep? Try rocking him in your arms or a cradle or pushing him up and down in the pram. At night, sleeping with their mothers is soothing for most babies.

■ Is he irritated by noise and people? Take him into a dark, quiet room.

3

■ Is he in pain? Check his clothing for tightness around his wrists, neck and ankles. A baby with nappy rash may cry if his nappy is wet or dirty.

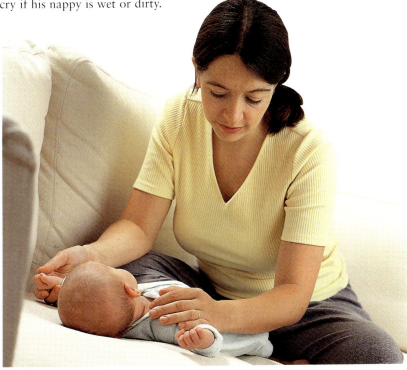

TRAVELLING

Breast milk is the best go-anywhere food, and breastfeeding means that, when you're away from home with your baby, you need no bottles, packs of milk, teats or worries about where you can make his feeds. You don't have to think about the milk going sour, or getting cold, or picking up bugs.

Your baby's milk is always there, at the right temperature. In addition, breastfeeding provides him with a familiar comfort when he's somewhere new and possibly confusing.

TIPS FOR BREASTFEEDING

Here are some tried and tested tips on taking your breastfed baby out and about with you.

■ A baby sling or carrier can make it possible to feed your baby when you are walking around with him – although it can take some practice to do this comfortably.

■ If you're not keen on people seeing what you're doing, a shawl or a throw placed around your shoulders can help you to be discreet.

■ If you prefer to go somewhere private and you can see no suitable mother and baby room, ask to use the staff restroom if you are in a shop or a shopping centre.

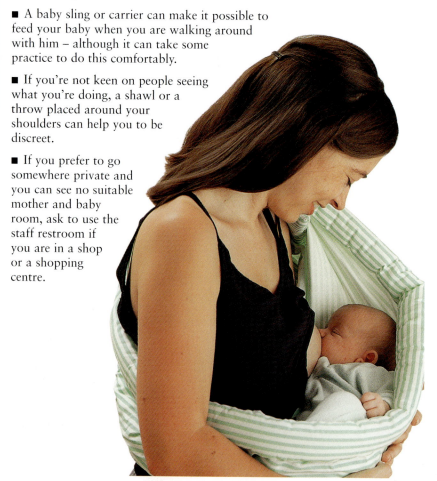

3

HOT WEATHER TIPS

If you go somewhere hot, be prepared for your baby to need more feeds in order to quench his thirst. There is normally no need to give water or other fluids to a healthy, thriving, breastfed baby who is fed unrestrictedly.

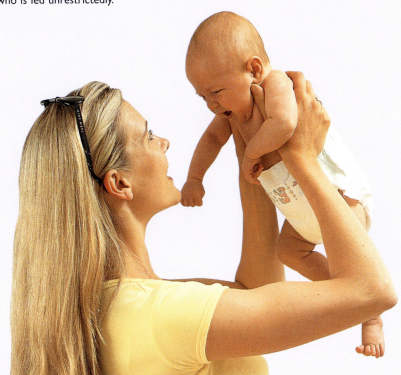

3

FEELING BRAVE?

If someone asks you to move, or to stop feeding, you can ask if they'd prefer to hear your baby cry loudly instead!

But remember, you may have no legally-protected right to breastfeed wherever you are (although you do have in some states in the USA), and if you're confronted you may have no option but to comply.

However, ask to speak to a superior and check out the company policy if it's a private building, or local authority policy in a public place. You may manage to get something changed, or else discover that no policy exists.

FLYING

When travelling on a plane, let your baby feed on take-off and landing to alleviate any pain in his ears from the change in air pressure. Sucking and swallowing is the easiest way for a baby, as well as an adult, to deal with this discomfort.

EXPRESSING BREAST MILK

The usual reason for expressing breast milk is to make it available (in a bottle or a cup) for your baby when you are not there. This may be because you are at work – in which event you may need to express every day – or because you want, or need, some time away from your baby occasionally, when you would need to express milk less regularly.

A few mothers have to express milk from the start, because their babies are unable to feed at the breast for some reason. These are babies with a severe cleft lip and/or palate; those who are born several weeks pre-term and can't coordinate sucking and swallowing (a skill which isn't present if the baby is very much pre-term); or who are too ill or weak to suck. Such babies may have to be tube fed with expressed breast milk (see pages 98–99 and 102–103).

Expressing is quite a complicated matter, and there is no 'one size fits all' set of solutions to everyone's situation. If you express often, you'll discover what works best for you by trial and error.

3

HOW OFTEN TO EXPRESS

If you are expressing instead of breastfeeding, you need to express at least as often as you'd expect your baby to feed. That way, your supply of breast milk is stimulated. For a young baby, you should aim to express at least 6–8 times in 24 hours, including at night. For an older baby – one of three or four months or more – who is being breastfed when you're with him, you should express every three to four hours. This means once or twice in the working day if you feed your baby last thing before you leave him, and first thing when you get back.

THE BEST TIME TO DO IT

This is up to you. Some women express immediately after a breastfeed. Some do it at the same time as their baby is feeding – with the pump at the breast the baby isn't on. Others do it between feeds. Find out what suits you best. You won't be 'stealing' milk the baby needs – expressing stimulates your breasts to make milk, so you are increasing your supply, not decreasing it.

KNOWING WHEN TO STOP

There's normally no point in spending more than about half an hour expressing; use both breasts and swap backward and forward if you find this is more productive. Some women get a reasonable yield in about 10 minutes and find it easier to stop and try again a little later if necessary.

You won't express very much at first. If your baby is very new, 5 or 10mls at a time is normal. Later on, if breastfeeding is well established, you may achieve 50mls or even 100mls at a time.

PUMPS OR HANDS?

Although a lot of women learn to express milk by hand and become very adept at it, a pump – electric or manual – is helpful. Your midwife or a breastfeeding counsellor can teach you how to use both methods.

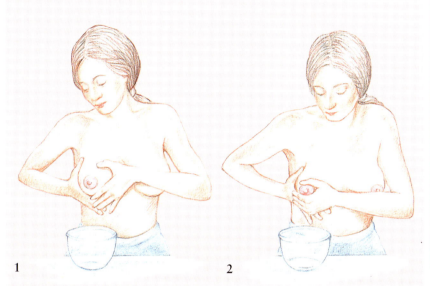

3

1

2

Support the breast in one hand and stroke steadily downward with the other. Then, 1, supporting the breast in your hand, with the thumb about

halfway down, stroke firmly toward the nipple. When you reach the areola, 2, press the thumb in and up and milk will flow from the nipple.

You can buy small mains- or battery-operated pumps. In some areas, you can hire a large electric one, or your hospital may lend you one if your baby is ill or pre-term.

Some pumps allow you to double pump, which means you can express both breasts at the same time.

Several good manually operated pumps are also available.

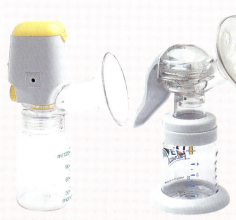

Battery-operated pump   Manually operated pump

HOW MUCH BREAST MILK MAKES A FEED?

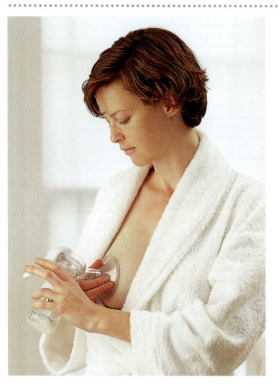

This is difficult! Babies differ so much. Tiny pre-term babies can take only a small amount – maybe a few drops at a time. Older, stronger babies take a lot more. A very rough rule of thumb is that a feed is something between 100mls and 200mls – with older babies taking more at any one time.

Most women find they need to express more than once to produce a whole feed, at least at first. But don't worry – the amount you can express is not an indication of how much you are capable of producing for your baby. Breasts respond better to a baby than to a pump or hands.

HOW DO I STORE EXPRESSED BREAST MILK?

Breast milk is safe in the fridge for 24 hours and in the freezer for 3 months. Sterilize anything you keep the milk in before you use it. Freeze breast milk in small quantities – ice cube trays are ideal. Small amounts defrost quickly, and you don't need to defrost more than you need at any one time.

Defrost the milk either by standing it in the fridge overnight or by standing the container in a jug of boiling water. The milk should be at body temperature when you give it to your baby – test a few drops on your wrist or the back of your hand to make sure that it is right for him.

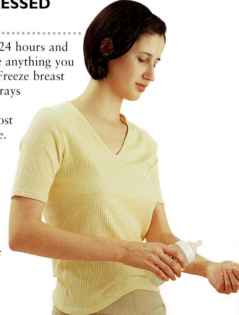

SOLVING BREASTFEEDING PROBLEMS

Breastfeeding is the natural way to feed your baby – but many women encounter problems that make it a challenge. However, almost every problem associated with breastfeeding can be resolved or, better, prevented.

Sometimes, mothers think their baby isn't getting enough milk, or that their milk supply isn't adequate – but we show that there are ways of checking this.

If there is something not quite right, fixing the breastfeeding so that it's effective, pain-free and happy for both mother and baby should be the first step. But only too often the step taken is to stop breastfeeding or to introduce formula milk instead of a breastfeed, or after it as a 'top-up'.

But, with persistence, most problems can be solved and you can manage to feed your baby breast milk alone.

4

NOT ENOUGH MILK?

The World Health Organization estimates that 98 per cent of women are physically capable of making sufficient breast milk to nourish their babies on that alone for at least six months. The remaining 2 per cent can be accounted for, at least in part, by factors such as illness or a physical difficulty with the mother or difficulty with the baby's sucking skills. Nevertheless, believing they have 'not enough milk' is a major reason why women give up breastfeeding.

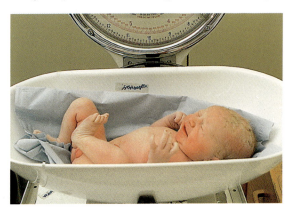

Lack of confidence in your milk supply can make you worry that you aren't feeding your baby well, and other people's comments about the value of breastfeeding can also create doubts in your mind.

A WELL-FED BABY

Knowing how to judge whether your baby is receiving enough breast milk for her needs is important. These are the signs of well-fed baby.

■ She is gaining weight satisfactorily. Your healthcare professionals can weigh your baby regularly to check this for you. Bear in mind that some babies don't gain weight at the same rate week after week, and that some will gain more slowly than others.

■ She latches on happily without too much fuss or struggle. Some babies may take a little while to master this skill.

■ She is producing wet and dirty nappies. After a few weeks, it is normal for some babies to produce a bowel motion only every few days. Others do it far more often than this. Constipation does not occur in fully breastfed babies (see page103).

■ She looks alert when she is awake.

■ She often asks for feeds. You may lose count of the number of times your baby is at the breast in 24 hours, but 12 or more times is normal in the early days and weeks (see pages 36–37). Babies who consistently have to be woken for feeds may simply lack the energy to ask for them.

4

IF SHE'S NOT GETTING ENOUGH

If you suspect that you may not be producing enough milk, here's what to do.

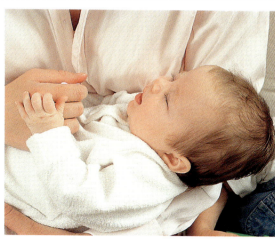

■ Ask someone who has some skill and expertise in helping women breastfeed to check the way your baby takes the breast and is positioned at the breast. It is not enough for them to check when your baby is already attached – the process of latching on is important, too (see pages 32–33).

■ Check the way your baby feeds. Is she sucking and swallowing happily? The pace of her sucking and swallowing may change, and it will probably slow down after the first minute or two. If there are a few sucks and swallows,

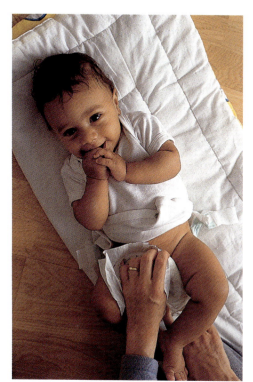

followed by the baby doing nothing but sleep at the breast, she may need to be woken up a little in order to get her to feed more. Change her nappy or remove some clothing.

4

■ Feed her more often. We have already seen that the more your baby feeds the more milk you'll make (see pages 44–45). Hold your baby close to you, so you can respond to her feeding cues more quickly.

■ Let your baby suck on the breast for as long as she seems to want – don't impose a time limit on her. Allow her to finish the first breast so that she can take the hind milk she needs. Then offer her the second breast. It's fine to offer 'three sides' at a feed, too, if your baby will take it. The stimulation will help to increase your milk supply.

MY BABY WON'T FEED

It can be very distressing for both you and your baby if she doesn't feed, and it can lead to a great deal of anxiety. Not all babies take to breastfeeding immediately, and then feed every time for as long as necessary without any complaints.

Sometimes, your baby may stay asleep, or fight at the breast, or come off after just a few sucks. There's a range of possible reasons why she is doing this.

IS IT A PROBLEM WITH LET DOWN?

The let down reflex, or milk ejection reflex, must take place in order for your baby to feed satisfactorily (see pages 26–29). It may be suggested to you that your baby can't get the let down to work or that your let down is 'failing'. And this may be offered as a possible reason why she shows signs of frustration or impatience at the breast.

In some ways this makes sense. After all, if the milk is in there, but the baby can't get at it, she will become cross, and then hungry. If the milk is not removed from the breast efficiently, this will affect your supply and, in time, your baby's growth.

4

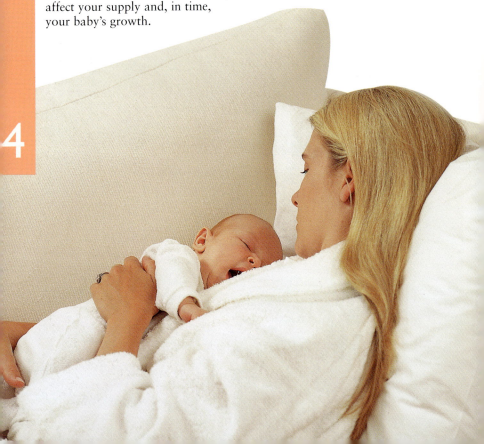

LET DOWN FAILURE

The truth is that let down is almost always reliable, except in very rare circumstances, and failure of let down is almost certainly diagnosed far more often than it actually happens. If your baby is well latched on – this might need to be checked (see pages 32–33) – and able to feed effectively, and you let her feed without taking her off before she has finished, your let down will function. In fact, when breastfeeding is well established you can get a let down without much help from your baby.

There are a number of let downs during most feeds, but you may not be aware of more than one or two, if that. You may feel a tingling or a sort of 'surge', and if your baby breaks off from the breast as a let down happens, you'll often see a surprisingly powerful spurt of milk from your nipple.

Let down in established breastfeeding happens as soon as the baby starts to suck, and sometimes even before then. You may find that you get a let down even by thinking about your baby, or hearing her cry. Or even hearing someone else's baby cry!

Just occasionally, some mothers suspect that a stressful situation can inhibit their let down. On some occasions they may be so stressed that they need to go somewhere quiet and relaxing in order to feed – and when they do, they calm down, their baby calms down, and the milk flows. Even more rarely, serious shock or very bad news can affect the let down. This is thought to be hormonal – but again it is normally temporary and resolves itself in the space of a feed or two.

IS YOUR LET DOWN TOO POWERFUL ?

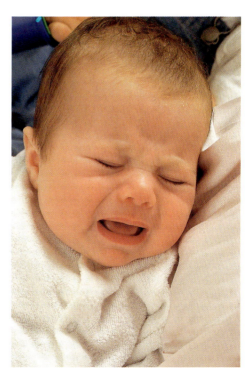

4

At the start of breastfeeding, a powerful let down can overwhelm a small baby, and she may come off the breast, spluttering and crying.

Normally, it is only a matter of time before she becomes more skilled at coping with your flow, and your supply settles down so that the milk doesn't spurt out so quickly.

In the meantime, it can be helpful if you express just a little of your milk before you put your young baby to the breast.

This will help to get a let down going so that it doesn't happen after your baby has taken only a few sucks and surprise her.

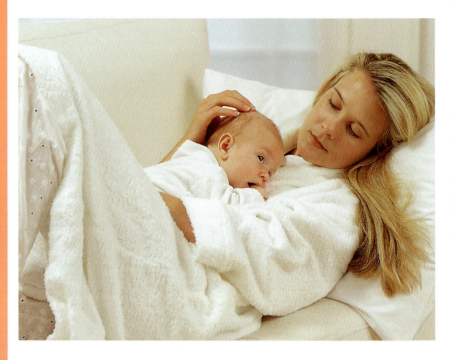

IS SHE TOO SLEEPY TO FEED?

Some medications used for pain during labour, such as diamorphine, are known to make babies sleepy after birth, and this can prevent them responding to the breast: they remain tight-lipped, with eyes closed. A long and tiring labour can have the same effect.

Give your baby time to get over the effect of any drugs and, in the meantime, give her lots of chances to be skin-to-skin with you, tucked up beside you in bed or in a chair. That will ensure that when she does flicker awake a little, you can respond. Just be gentle and don't fight with her or try to push her on to your breast.

Open her clothing, bath her, change her nappy – do anything that might wake her up a bit without upsetting her.

You can express a little colostrum by hand into a cup or syringe and place a few drops on your baby's lips to tempt her. Help her lap up some colostrum from a cup if she goes longer than a day or two without feeding. But don't do this instead of following all the other suggestions; do it alongside them.

DOES SHE REALLY WANT TO FEED?

Older babies, and some younger ones, want or need to stay at the breast for only a very short time. They get what they need and then want to come off. This is especially the case with babies who are starting to take an interest in the world about them. In addition, you may be very efficient at making and letting down the milk, so everything is over in a few minutes. Don't be tempted to try to force your baby to stay on longer – she'll get cross.

IS SHE ILL?

Don't think your new baby is 'good' if she goes a long time between feeds – more than three or four hours – other than just occasionally. She could be poorly, and dehydrated and lethargic as a result. Babies who are failing to thrive may also get so sleepy that they don't have the energy to wake for feeds. Seek medical advice.

Any change in feeding pattern that means your baby feeds much less than before can be cause for concern. She could have an ear infection, for example. Very occasionally a baby who is not interested in feeding may have a congenital problem, such as a heart defect (see pages 100–101), so it is always important to have your baby checked over by a paediatrician if this is a persistent situation.

IS SHE ON STRIKE?

Nursing strike is something that can happen at any time, but with gentle persuasion most babies get over it. For some reason, a previously happy breastfeeding baby refuses the breast and cries instead. If your baby is not ill, hold her a lot, at night as well as during the day, and try to feed her when she is dozy and less aware. See your doctor or health visitor if this persists.

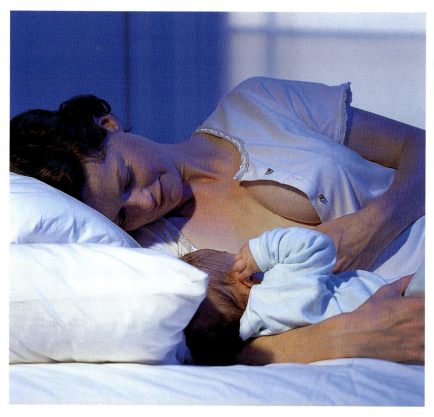

4

SORE NIPPLES

There's no doubt that sore nipples can cause a great deal of misery. The nipple is one of the most sensitive areas of the human body: a graze or a blister on it can quickly become a crack as the baby sucks – and this is very painful.

Some tenderness at the beginning of breastfeeding is so common that it is probably normal – though this is controversial, and not everyone agrees. The tenderness should get better as time goes on, not worse. If a nipple is truly painful, the chances are that your baby is not latched on in a way that allows her to feed without your nipple becoming sore.

Most frequently, the nipple isn't far enough into the baby's mouth, so it rubs against the edge of the baby's hard palate. Sometimes the baby's jaws have clamped down so hard on the nipple – instead of the baby scooping in breast tissue with her tongue – that the pressure actually abrades and damages the skin.

If this is the case, it is essential to change the way your baby takes the breast so that she comes on and stays on in a way that is pain-free, and which allows her to feed effectively (see pages 32–35). Changing your baby's position, and the way you sit when feeding, can sometimes help.

OTHER CAUSES OF SORE NIPPLES

Sore nipples can also be caused by:

■ thrush (see pages 74–75)

■ dermatitis. You may be allergic to soap powder or fabric softener, for example. Just occasionally, some mothers react to their baby's saliva when they go onto solid food

■ eczema or psoriais. These skin conditions can develop on almost any part of the body

USING CREAMS

Little research has been done on using creams to heal sore nipples, but some mothers feel that they speed up healing and soothe the tender areas. Use a nipple cream if you like, but don't use one instead of checking your baby's position and attachment.

USING BREASTMILK

Some mothers find it soothing to put expressed breast milk on their nipples. There's no scientific proof that it is beneficial, but it's worth a try, since you can be sure there will no side effects.

NIPPLE SHIELDS

Experienced midwives and other breastfeeding supporters have mixed feelings about using nipple shields (thin rubber covers that go over the nipples to protect them if they are sore or cracked).

Nipple shields have their drawbacks. First, they can teach a baby to suck in a different way, with the result that the baby becomes hooked on them and unable to feed without them. Second, they cut down the rate at which the milk is transferred to the baby, probably because the breast is not stimulated in quite the same way. This can result in poor weight gain and failing milk supply. However, if the baby can latch on to the shield correctly and take a lot of breast into her mouth, it seems there are fewer problems. Shields do need to be used with caution, and with the support of someone who understands their use.

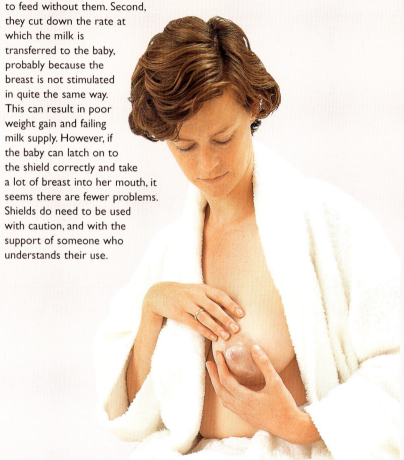

4

INVERTED NIPPLES

True inverted nipples look like a little dimple, rather than protruding, and can make it harder for your baby to latch on. However, successful breastfeeding is still possible, although you may need more patience, and your baby may need more practice. There are some techniques that might help evert them, but the only techniques that have been examined by a proper trial have not been shown to be any more successful than doing nothing.

MASTITIS

This is the term used to describe inflammation of the breast, a condition that is quite common. However, if treated correctly, it's not serious, or a threat to breastfeeding, or harmful to you or your baby.

Mastitis develops for two possible reasons.

The less common cause is an infection entering the breast, sometimes via bacteria in the baby's nose.

The other, far more common cause, is inflammation resulting from a blockage in one of the milk ducts. This happens if milk gets stuck in the duct and remains there. The milk then starts to leak into the surrounding tissue, and this produces a classic inflammatory response in the body, which recognizes that the milk shouldn't be where it is. A red patch develops on your breast, as extra blood rushes to the site, and you may be able to feel a lump there.

Your breast seems more susceptible to infection in this state, although we don't yet fully understand the mechanism of mastitis and infection. Some women start to feel flu-like symptoms, and it can be painful to touch the breast and to feed your baby.

Some experts distinguish between a blocked duct as such and the mastitis that results from it, but the distinction is rather arbitrary – once you're aware of a blocked duct it's already inflamed, and you may as well term it mastitis and take appropriate action.

SELF-HELP FOR MASTITIS

Give yourself 12 to 24 hours to deal with mastitis yourself.

■ Feed the baby first on the affected side, when she is most hungry, to encourage the duct to drain.

■ Massage the affected breast, very gently and for some time, either in the shower or the bath, which seems to help the milk to flow. Otherwise you can gently massage the breast during the feed.

■ Try feeding your baby with the breast hanging down into her mouth, to see if gravity can help shift the blockage.

■ Applying warmth to the affected part of your breast seems to help, too. Try using a warmed cloth or cover a hot water bottle with a cloth or small towel and hold it against your breast.

■ Feed your baby frequently, giving her every chance to help drain the blocked duct and so clear up the inflammation by her sucking.

4

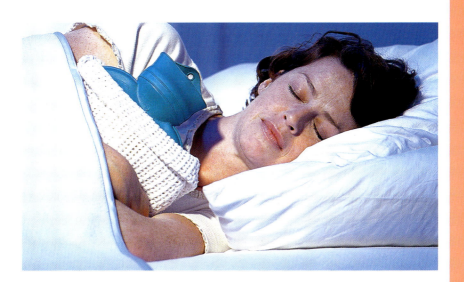

IF IT DOESN'T GET BETTER

■ Ask your doctor or midwife for advice if the mastitis persists after 24 hours.

■ If you're prescribed antibiotics (which deal with inflammation and help prevent infection), remind the doctor that you need medication which is compatible with breastfeeding

■ Disregard any advice to stop feeding. This is the last thing you should do and can make the problem worse, since you will continue to make milk for a while. You will feel even more uncomfortable as a result, and some people think that this could increase your risk of developing a breast abscess.

AVOIDING MASTITIS

Decrease the risk of developing mastitis by:

■ checking that you're not wearing a bra or clothing that could press down on a duct and 'kink' it to prevent it from draining.

■ feeding as often as your baby wants.

■ not leaving too long between feeds. For instance, ducts can become blocked the first time the baby goes through the night without feeding.

4

BREAST ABSCESS

Fortunately, breast abscesses are very rare. An abscess is an untreated infection in the breast, a collection of pus that gathers on the affected part of the breast, often after an attack of mastitis. You will know you have one because a swollen area develops on the breast, which may be red.

The abscess will sometimes respond to large doses of antibiotics, but if it doesn't, it will need surgical treatment. A tube is inserted and the abscess is either aspirated (sucked out) or drained. You will need a local anaesthetic and, depending on where the incision is, your baby may not be able to feed on that side until the incision has completely healed.

IS BREASTFEEDING BEST?

Many women who start breastfeeding stop before they plan to – usually because it just hasn't worked out for them. They stop with regret, and after some thought, because they come to the conclusion that they, and possibly their baby, will be happier if they introduce formula.

IS GIVING UP THE ONLY OPTION?

Think about what's making it hard for you. If you had planned to breastfeed, and will experience some regret if you stop, see if you can overcome the problem first. Common reasons mothers have for giving up are:

■ 'Breastfeeding is such a tie…I miss going out without the baby.'

Once breastfeeding is established, you can leave a bottle of expressed breast milk for your baby for a carer to offer if she needs it. Or, if this isn't possible, the occasional bottle of formula is an option – this is better for your baby than no breastfeeding at all (see pages 86–87).

■ 'It is such a struggle. I have had so many problems, and it is just not working out. I want to start enjoying feeding and stop dreading it.'

Seek proper sympathetic and knowledgeable help and information (see pages 76–78). There may be some difficulties ahead, and breastfeeding that's difficult may not become easy overnight. But unless you're confident that the advice you've had so far fully supports your desire to breastfeed, there may well be other options.

■ 'It's gone so badly. I've given my baby so many bottles now. She has one after most feeds – and I think it's time to call it a day.'

If you think your milk supply is diminishing as a result of giving bottles, it may be possible to increase it, but you need to be very committed (see page 111).

■ 'I feel so selfish. I feel it's me wanting to breastfeed and my baby wanting to bottle feed. She always settles better after a bottle feed.'

Your baby will benefit healthwise from successful breastfeeding, but bottle feeding is clearly more satisfying for her, in the short term, than a struggle with breastfeeding. Babies may settle to sleep better after a bottle feed simply because they become fuller more quickly. Working on the breastfeeding may help you to achieve the same result without a bottle. Don't feel selfish – you have your baby's long-term interests at heart as well as your own desire to breastfeed.

4

DECIDING TO STOP

If you do decide to stop, see pages 108–109 for how to cope with your feelings, and how to make up your mind as to whether now is the right time for you and/or your baby to make the switch to formula. Remember, it's your decision and you must do what you really want to.

WHAT PEOPLE MAY SAY TO YOU

When you are in a quandary about whether to persist with breastfeeding, you will get plenty of comments that may make you waver, such as:

■ 'Don't make a rod for your own back – you're making yourself so distressed, for nothing.'

■ 'Formula is just as good and nourishing as breast milk nowadays.'

■ 'I bottle fed all of my children, and they have turned out fine.'

■ 'If only you'd bottle feed – I could do more to help you.'

BENEFITS TO YOU

Would you feel less tired if you stopped breastfeeding?

Breastfeeding is not in itself physically tiring, and you have to sit down or lie down to do it. In addition, the very act of breastfeeding helps you secrete a hormone that aids relaxation. And if you stop, you have to balance the 'effort' of breastfeeding with the work involved in the daily preparation of bottles of formula.

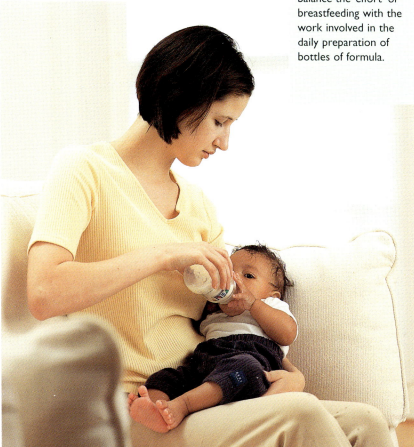

4

THRUSH

Thrush – or candida to give it the medical name – is an infection caused by the fungus *Candida albicans*, which can exist almost anywhere in the body.

Many women suffer from occasional bouts of vaginal thrush, which is characterized by an itchy, sometimes sore, vagina and vulva – with a discharge like cottage cheese if the infection takes hold.

Thrush can also affect your nipples, and even the ducts inside your breasts. The warm, sugary environment of the nipple and the milk ducts creates a perfect situation for thrush to thrive.

SIGNS OF INFECTION IN YOURSELF

Suspect thrush if you have sore, cracked, itchy or sensitive nipples and any of the following apply as well.

■ Your nipples became sore after a period of happy feeding.

■ Despite a change of position or improved latching on, your sore nipples don't improve.

■ You have had a course of antibiotics. These make you more susceptible to candida, since they reduce your body's ability to combat fungal infection.

■ You have had vaginal thrush. If this is the case, the fungus can be transferred to your baby during birth, or later on if your hands are not properly washed.

■ You have pain in the breast. Typically, mothers describe this as a shooting or radiating pain, during and/or after the feed.

SIGNS OF INFECTION IN YOUR BABY

Your baby may or may not have thrush inside her mouth. This will appear as a collection of white or creamy patches, on her tongue, gums or inside her cheeks, which don't rub off, or else come away, leaving raw patches behind.

If these are present, you can be pretty sure that your baby is suffering from thrush. It can sometimes mean that her mouth is so sore that she feeds with difficulty and seems unsettled, although some babies seem to be unaffected in this way.

It appears that mothers and babies can pass thrush backward and forward between them. As a result, if either you or your baby is affected, you will both need treatment. Don't think that if you are infected and your baby has no symptoms she does not need to be treated.

TREATING THRUSH

If you suspect that either you or your baby has thrush, see your doctor, who can confirm it and prescribe anti-fungal medication for both of you.

For your baby, the treatment might be

■ Gel

with anti-fungal medication, applied with a fingertip to the baby's mouth.

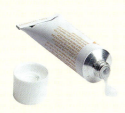

■ Drops

with anti-fungal medication, which must be swallowed.

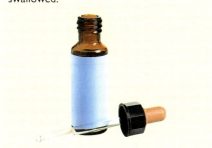

For you, the treatment might be

■ Cream

with anti-fungal medication, applied with a finger to the nipples.

■ Tablets or capsules

with anti-fungal medication, taken by mouth. This treatment is used for thrush which affects the milk ducts. The evidence is that a fairly long course of medication is needed – up to 14 days. The pain may not go away for 10 days, so you need to be patient. However, many women start to feel a difference sooner than this.

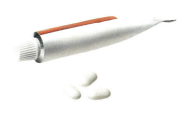

4

HOW TO PREVENT THRUSH SPREADING

The usual rules for hygiene apply.

■ Use a separate towel for each household member, so that infection doesn't get passed on in this way.

■ Anything your baby has in her mouth – such as a dummy, a bottle teat or a teething ring – needs to be sterilized for 20 minutes in boiling water. This seems to be more effective at killing thrush than sterilizing fluid or tablets. It's not known if steam sterilizing is effective.

■ If you use a pump to express milk, boil the pump parts that come into contact with your milk.

WHERE TO GET HELP

However you feed, when you're a new mother, you need friends, family and the chance to have some adult conversation from time to time. Your baby may be the best thing that's ever happened to you, but there's no doubt that she can't supply everything you need in terms of company, stimulation and entertainment. And if you're breastfeeding, you may need something more specific as well – the encouragement and help of people who know how it is done.

FRIENDS WHO ARE BREASTFEEDING

Research shows that having friends who breastfeed is a real source of support, and that mothers with such friends breastfeed for longer.

Ask your midwife or health visitor if there are any other mothers with young babies living locally. You may be near a peer counselling scheme, or be able to attend a breastfeeding support group. Both these offer mother-to-mother support and friendship.

If you're going through a bad patch, or a tiring few days, it's a great comfort to find someone who tells you, 'That happened to me – and this is what I did, which helped.' Bear in mind that what works for one person doesn't necessarily work for everyone – but the support you get from people who are keen to breastfeed, and the boost to your confidence from seeing people at a later stage of breastfeeding, is invaluable.

4

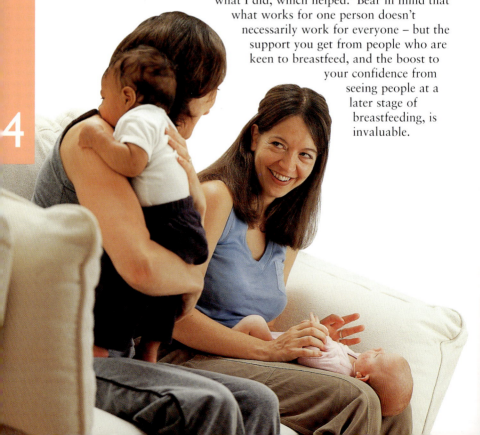

PROFESSIONAL SUPPORT

Some health professionals are a great source of support. They recognize the importance of breastfeeding, and how your feelings can affect your success.

■ Midwives and health visitors have all had some training in helping women breastfeed, but some of them are not as up to date as others, although this situation is changing. If you aren't happy with the advice or information you receive, ask to speak to someone else, or ask if there are any alternative approaches.

■ Doctors are not normally experts on everyday breastfeeding, although some are well informed and supportive. You cannot assume that doctors have studied breastfeeding at medical school, and their knowledge sometimes depends on their own experience of infant feeding – but that can be misleading. Allowing personal experience to fill the gap in training can lead to erroneous advice. Again, if you feel unhappy with the advice you get, ask for a second opinion.

LAY SUPPORTERS

There are several organizations that train mothers who have breastfed to enable them to support and encourage other mothers. These women may be called counsellors or supporters.The training programmes focus on supporting the mother and helping her feel empowered to make her own feeding choices. Counsellors won't try to force you to breastfeed, or to continue breastfeeding if you don't want to.

Your health visitor or midwife can let you know of counsellors in your area, or you can contact a central number and ask for local representatives. Some organizations run groups; others offer mainly one-to-one support. Most counsellors offer telephone counselling, and these days e-mail counselling is becoming more common.

You may need to see a counsellor – especially if you have problems with positioning and attaching your baby, which is difficult to discuss over the phone. Often it may not be a question of finding a hint or a tip to 'solve' your problem. Instead you will be encouraged to talk through options, to work out what course of action will suit you. This will be backed up by a good knowledge of how breastfeeding works physiologically, so your counsellor will be able to explain the likely impact on your breastfeeding if you choose one option rather than another.

So, saying to a counsellor, 'Should I give my baby a bottle?' will not bring the answer yes or no. You'll be asked to explore why you think this might help, what effect it might have, and what the outcome might be.

4

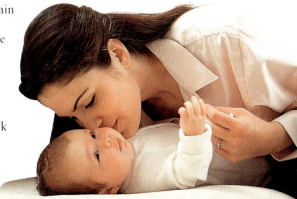

POST-NATAL DEPRESSION

This is a condition that affects an estimated 12 to 15 per cent of new mothers, and many more mothers have times when they feel lonely, distressed, anxious and isolated.

If you think you may be suffering from post-natal depression, you will need extra help and support from those around you. But don't think you have to stop breastfeeding. For some women, breastfeeding is the one positive aspect of parenting that sustains them through this difficult time. For others, it seems to be no more than just one more demand on them that makes them feel guilty and lacking in confidence.

If you want to continue breastfeeding while undergoing treatment for post-natal depression, tell your doctor. She may be able to prescribe safe medication. If you need to be in hospital for treatment, aim to go there with your baby. Even if you are too ill to care for your baby, staying close and building your relationship is easier if your baby is with you for at least some of the time. See also pages 104–105.

4

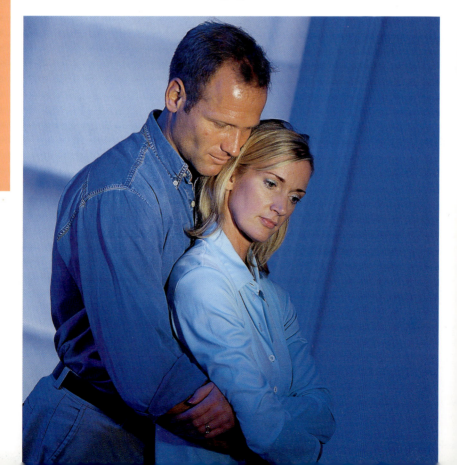

BREASTFEEDING AN OLDER BABY

You can go on breastfeeding your baby for as long as you both want to do it. But when you do decide that you want to stop, you will want to do so in a way that doesn't distress or confuse your baby. There are gentle ways to wean, and here we tell you how to combine breastfeeding with solid foods, and when to start.

We also discuss the pros and cons of introducing bottles, and explain how breastfeeding changes as your baby gets older.

Although most mothers start by breastfeeding, it's a minority who continue beyond the first few weeks. This is a pity because frequently it's soon after this time that breastfeeding becomes a relaxed, everyday relationship – you're more confident and your baby is often quite an expert. And this is the time that many mothers think 'I'm glad I stayed with it – it's definitely worth it!'

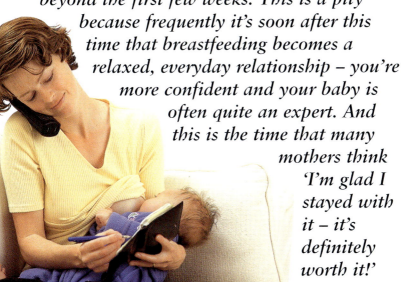

5

ADDING SOLID FOOD

Current recommendations are that most babies are ready to have solid food – the term 'solid' means any food that's not milk – at between four and six months of age. Some experts feel that where there is a family history of allergies, babies should be at least six months old.

WHEN TO INTRODUCE SOLID FOOD

You might think about introducing solids if your baby is at least four months old, and the following apply.

■ He is showing an interest in the food on other people's plates, perhaps reaching out to touch it.

■ He can pick up objects and suck them to investigate them more closely.

■ He enjoys a few offerings of solid food when he's sitting on your lap. Choose a time that's convenient to you. You may be going back to work, and you'd like your childminder to give him a solid meal plus a drink in the middle of the day, instead of having to express breast milk.

   Don't complicate life by introducing solid foods if you're planning to go on holiday – your baby can wait. First solids are a way to help your baby get used to different tastes and textures. Breast milk is more nourishing for him.

THE FIRST FOODS

You don't have to buy anything special for your baby. There are foods which are suitable for your baby from the very beginning and which you can share with him. Mash, sieve or puree the following foods to get rid of any lumps and don't add any seasoning, salt or sugar.

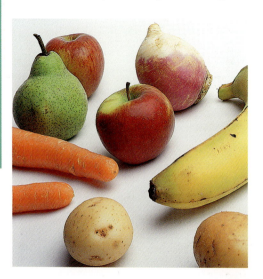

■ Cooked potato

■ Cooked swede or turnip

■ Cooked carrot

■ Soft dessert pear, peeled

■ Soft, dessert apple, peeled

■ Banana

   Whatever you choose for your baby's first taste of solid food, offer it in tiny quantities at first. Healthy babies know their own appetites, and forcing the issue only makes mealtimes a source of frustration and anxiety.

5

HOW OFTEN SHOULD I GIVE SOLIDS?

Once a day is fine for solids at first. It can be before, after or even during your baby's breastfeed – do what suits you. As you build up your baby's repertoire, you can begin to time feeding solid foods to coincide with your normal mealtimes. Some babies take three months or more to build up to eating breakfast, lunch and tea; others get there very quickly.

FOODS TO INTRODUCE LATER

Some foods are difficult for a young digestive system to cope with, and they may be linked to the development of food allergies or intolerance if they are introduced too early. They are fine to give to your baby after he has become accustomed to some basic, simple foods.

Introduce these foods later.

■ Cereals containing gluten. Gluten is present in wheat and in any foods containing wheat. These include most flour products, including bread.

■ Eggs. Offer the well-cooked yolk at about six months, then the white when your baby is about eight months old.

■ Citrus fruits.

■ Cheeses.

■ Nuts.

■ Meat and fish.

FINGER FOODS

Lots of foods can be offered as finger foods. Simply cut or slice them into a size your baby can hold and manoeuvre easily, while chewing, gnawing or sucking them. Some babies prefer eating in this way this to spoon-feeding.

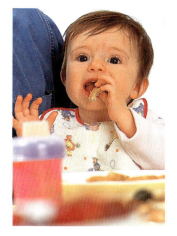

Warning!

Always stay with your baby when he's feeding himself in case he chokes.

5

PREPARING FOODS

Mashing with a fork is usually all that is needed for most foods, even for a young baby. If you feed all pureed food, some babies will get so used to its smooth texture that they start to resist anything that's not totally free of lumps.

HEALTHY BABY FOODS

After they are about six months old, babies need more calories for energy and extra iron, which comes from cereals, dairy produce, eggs, meat, fish and pulses.

Your baby also needs to practise his social skills, and joining in meals with other people provides a great opportunity for this.

LITTLE AND OFTEN

It's normal for babies to eat or drink several times a day, including meals and snacks, without taking much at any one sitting. Babies need calorie-dense foods, and they benefit from the fat-soluble vitamins present in whole yoghurt, full-fat cheeses and other products. So stick to full-fat dairy foods for your baby. Remember: the healthy advice to choose low-fat foods is directed at adults – not babies and young children.

Choose unsweetened foods; relying on sugary foods can give your baby a sweet tooth, which is bad for his dental health.

A NINE-MONTH-OLD BABY NEEDS

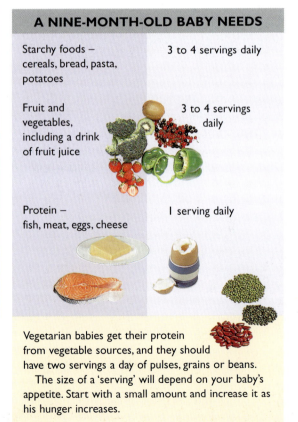

Starchy foods – cereals, bread, pasta, potatoes — 3 to 4 servings daily

Fruit and vegetables, including a drink of fruit juice — 3 to 4 servings daily

Protein – fish, meat, eggs, cheese — 1 serving daily

Vegetarian babies get their protein from vegetable sources, and they should have two servings a day of pulses, grains or beans.

The size of a 'serving' will depend on your baby's appetite. Start with a small amount and increase it as his hunger increases.

PACKETS, TINS AND JARS

Bought baby foods are easy, safe and convenient to use.

They are made without artificial additives, but read the label to avoid any that are highly sweetened, and those with a large water content. Remember, the main ingredient of any packaged food is listed first on the label.

The biggest disadvantages of bought baby foods are that they are very expensive to use all the time and that they tend to be smooth, so a baby doesn't get used to foods with different textures.

ADDING VITAMINS

Ask your health visitor or doctor about vitamin supplements. Older babies and toddlers whose diets are good, and who have the chance to go outside every day, don't need supplements – vitamin D can be processed by the body through access to sunlight.

THINGS YOUR BABY CAN'T YET EAT

Avoid whole nuts (babies can easily choke on them).

Salted foods are not suitable; they can make a baby very thirsty, and unless he is given adequate liquids severe dehydration can occur. Dehydration is very dangerous in young babies.

True food allergy is unusual, but it does exist. You should get a proper diagnosis if you suspect your child reacts adversely to the same food each time you give it. Serious reactions need medical treatment straightaway.

YOUR BABY AND FAMILY MEALS

After six months, your baby can join in more and more with the family meals. Seat him at the table in a high chair or on your lap. You may need to give him his main evening meal earlier than you have yours – a baby can't wait until seven o'clock for his tea, unless he has a substantial snack in the afternoon. And some babies are asleep by this time. Similarly, some older babies want an early lunch – at about 11 to 11.30 am – after which they will have a post-lunch nap. You'll find it's easier if you are fairly flexible about mealtimes and expect your baby's routine to change from time to time.

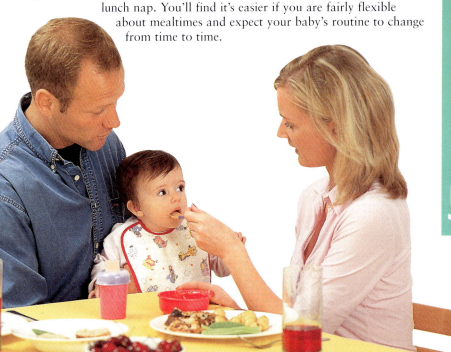

5

LATER BREASTFEEDING

As time goes on, don't expect breastfeeding to feel the same to you. At first, prolactin 'makes' the milk, as we saw on pages 26–29. But tests show that prolactin levels in the blood fall throughout the first six months after the birth. At some point during the first year they're back to normal, even if you're fully breastfeeding.

Breast milk is then produced under a different stimulus. It is made without prolactin, simply because it is taken from the breasts by your baby. This is called the 'autocrine', or 'self-driven', response, as opposed to the 'endocrine', or hormone-driven, response of the first days, weeks and months.

The exact biochemistry of this change is not fully understood, but it seems that the milk-production line gets to a stage where there is always milk available for your baby, and more is made as and when he sucks – without the round-the-clock extra production that leads to round-the-clock full breasts.

The same principle of 'supply and demand' is still crucial – the more your baby sucks, the more milk will be made for him. But the production line does not shut down if your baby goes rather longer between feeds, as many do when they have solid food, or if they sleep for longer periods, or if they spend time in a nursery or with a childminder.

'I'VE RUN OUT OF MILK!'

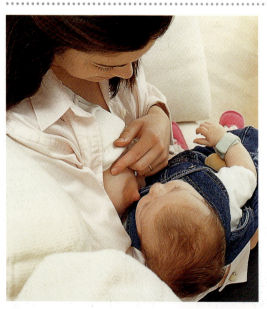

This cry is seldom true. Don't worry if you find your breasts getting softer and 'emptier' feeling as your baby gets older. This doesn't mean you can't produce what he wants. You're just not storing it – it's made on tap at the time of asking.

The flexibility of the system means that if your baby goes off solid food, or becomes ill, or needs extra milk for whatever reason and comes to your breast more often than before, or starts waking again at night, you can make more milk for him.

5

IT'S A FAST-FOOD OUTLET

How does this instant production function? It helps to imagine that you're the manager of a brand new fast-food restaurant.

At first you don't know how many burgers you will sell at any one time. To make sure you have enough, you ask your staff to make more burgers than you think you might need – so even if you get a rush, there will be some burgers there. Your staff are inexperienced, and they need a 'cushion' of extra burgers to ensure they don't run out and disappoint anyone.

After a while, your staff get pretty good, and quick. They don't need a 'cushion' to tide them over busy times. They can make burgers as the customers want them, and the more they sell, the more they make. They make them instantly, as soon as they're ordered, with only a few 'spares' at a time. But if you get an unexpected rush – no problem!

Your staff just work a little faster to respond, and soon start supplying the extras, as they're wanted.

This is almost exactly how your breastfeeding operates as you and your baby work together to become an experienced manager and customer.

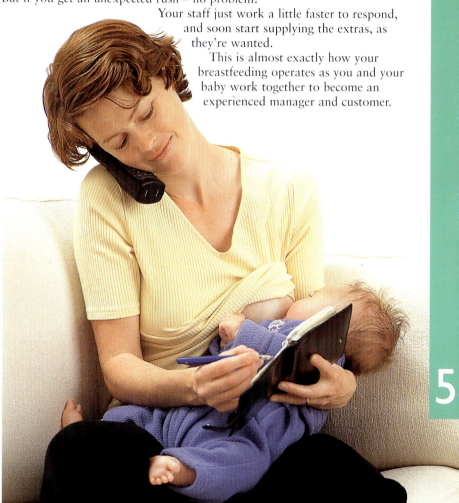

5

BREAST VERSUS BOTTLE

You may hear the warning that introducing bottles to a breastfed baby means less stimulation of the breast milk supply – and so less breast milk. A baby who takes a bottle instead of coming to the breast is likely to miss out on a breastfeed. If it's a bottle of formula, it may take longer to digest than breast milk, and so the gap between his breastfeeds is longer. If this happens more than just very occasionally, your body will respond by making less breast milk. However, in practice, it's a lot more complicated than that.

THE SUPPLY OF BREAST MILK

The supply of breast milk is adaptable and does not depend forever on the baby being given nothing else – but it is important to realize that the only safe time to introduce bottles is once breastfeeding is well established.

Not a lot of research has been done, but we do know that giving bottles during the first weeks is associated with giving up breastfeeding completely a few weeks later. But that could be, at least partly, because the bottles are introduced into a situation where there are already problems.

It may also depend on what is in the bottles. Some mothers give expressed breast milk in the bottle, and not formula. This means that the breasts have had the stimulation of the milk being expressed, so the bottle does not actually take the place of a breastfeed. So, even early on, this has probably less impact on the breast milk supply.

As the baby gets older, you can, with care, start using bottles of formula as a matter of convenience – although the later you leave it, the better, and the fewer bottles, the better.

HEALTH BENEFITS OF BREASTFEEDING

But what about the health benefits of breastfeeding? Is a partially breastfed baby less well-protected?

Some health benefits – protection against allergy and respiratory illness, for example – seem to depend on giving nothing but breast milk (defined as 'exclusive breastfeeding') for at least the first three to four months. The protection afforded by breast milk appears to be what the experts call 'dose related'. A smaller 'dose' of breast milk reduces the protection – but doesn't wipe it out.

It's true that some research indicates that a vulnerable baby may be sensitized by even one bottle of formula, and may develop a food or other form of allergy. But the majority of studies conclude that while full breastfeeding is best, some breastfeeding is a lot better than none at all.

5

HOW TO INTRODUCE FORMULA

If you have decided you want to combine bottles and breastfeeding:

■ Wait, if you can, until your baby is at least two months old (an arbitrary age but, for most mothers, breastfeeding is reliable by then).

■ Consider using expressed breast milk instead of formula.

Experience suggests that, on average, the breast-milk-production line needs regular stimulation for five to six months before it can survive on fewer than about five or six feeds or expressions a day – so don't mix breastfeeding and formula feeding too often, too soon.

NIPPLE CONFUSION

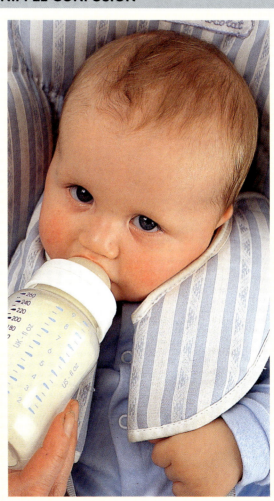

The difficulty encountered when the baby appears to forget how to breastfeed, after experiencing the different sucking technique needed with the bottle, is known as nipple confusion. In addition, dummies (pacifiers) can satisfy a baby's need to suck, leading them to spend less time on the breast (see pages 42–43).

Nipple confusion is a controversial issue. Some experts feel babies can do both, and it's only when there's a problem with breastfeeding that the baby starts to refuse to suck at the breast after having been given a bottle. It does seem that when breastfeeding has been going well, it can be resumed more easily.

For information on how to help your baby get used to a bottle, see pages 90–91.

5

FEEDING A TODDLER

Throughout the world, and throughout history, it has been normal for babies to be breastfed into toddlerhood and beyond.

Anthropologists have studied communities where breastfeeding is common, where bottles are rare if not unknown, and where babies and mothers sleep next to each other at night. For instance, in Mali, in West Africa – to take one example of many – the usual age of weaning from the breast is three or four.

In the West, seeing a child breastfed to this age or beyond is very unusual. It does happen, but mostly privately, and often at night. Sometimes, the decision to breastfeed, beyond the six months or a year seen as usual in our society, isn't really a conscious one – it just happens in the absence of a decision to wean. The baby and the mother carry on with breastfeeding because neither wish to stop, or wish to take action to encourage stopping.

5

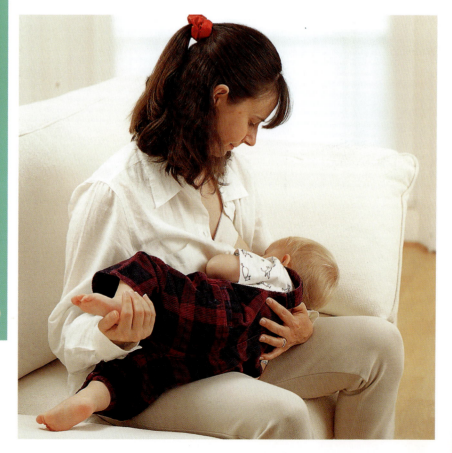

IS IT A GOOD THING?

Breastfeeding means that there is always a soothing way your child can be comforted, or helped to relax in order to get to sleep at night, and you always have something your child will take if he's ill. This can be important, since a poorly child needs fluid but will often reject it.

Working mothers find it a good way to 'connect' after a day spent apart from their child.

IT'S RELAXING FOR BOTH MOTHER AND CHILD

A child who is taking other foods won't depend on breast milk in the same way as a baby does – but breast milk has a role to play, since its quality is never in doubt. And your child will get nutritious food and drink with breast milk.

HOW DOES A TODDLER FEED?

Typically, toddlers feed in short bursts, with occasional longer feeds when tired. If you have left the pace and timing of feeds to your child, you may feed very often. If not, your toddler may have become used to breastfeeds at mealtimes, or when going to sleep, so it's only a few times each day, and maybe at night.

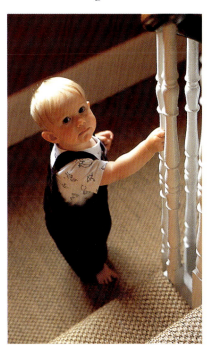

On the other hand, toddlers start to assert their own preferences as they get older, and they can start to ask for feeds outside this routine. You may have to decide whether to accept this, or gradually insist on feeds only at set times – say, once in the morning and once in the evening. It's up to you.

Sometimes, mothers decide to wean because they start to feel pressed to feed more often – and they don't want to have a struggle with their child. So they wean before it becomes a wrench that upsets the child.

5

OTHERS' REACTIONS

There may be people in your circle who think it's odd or mad to breastfeed beyond the baby stage – and for the sake of peace you may want to encourage your older toddler not to crawl under your jumper and help himself in company. However, toddlers and young children quickly learn when they can and can't breastfeed, and they seem to accept it very easily, as long as there are times when they know they can.

GOING BACK TO WORK

You don't need to give up breastfeeding your baby just because you are going back to work if you want to continue.

WHAT YOU CAN DO

■ Mix breastfeeding and bottle feeding – giving your baby the breast when you are together and leaving formula for your baby's carer to give to him when you are not there.

■ Express at work and possibly at home, which allows you to leave expressed breast milk (EBM) for your baby to be given by bottle or in a cup.

■ Change your working hours to allow you to visit your baby to feed him. Expressing maintains the milk supply, and reduces the discomfort of full breasts, and it ensures your baby has exclusively breast milk or more breast milk than formula.

Electric pumps are an easy way to express milk. The low-tech alternative is hand-expression. Once you have the knack, it can be almost as good as using an electric pump (see pages 58–59).

If you decide to mix breast and bottle, see pages 86–87.

TEACHING YOUR BABY TO TAKE A BOTTLE

Getting a baby who's a dedicated breastfeeder to take a bottle is occasionally a problem. Beyond the age of five or six months, don't persist if your baby is reluctant to accept a bottle – you can give the formula or expressed milk in a spouted cup instead.

A younger baby isn't able to manage a cup, so he should be introduced to bottle feeding and given a few practice bottles before you return to work – but ideally not by you. A baby can become understandably bewildered if their mother offers this strange plastic and rubber thing instead of the familiar

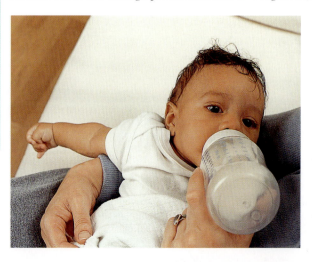

breast. Instead, allow your carer to offer the bottle. It is best to do this when your baby is not very hungry or cross.

If you give a bottle, be patient. You may have to give a breastfeed first, and then the bottle, sneaking in the teat when your baby is no longer feeling too hungry.

5

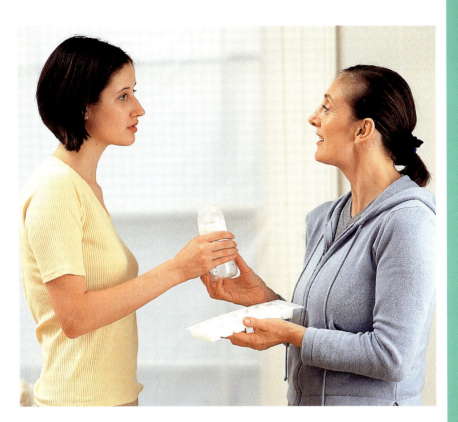

EXPRESSING AT WORK

An increasing number of employers are developing breastfeeding friendly policies. It's actually economic to do so. Breastfed babies are less likely to fall sick, so their mothers need less time off.

You need somewhere clean and private to express – the toilets are not suitable – and your employer should allow you to have a pleasant clean place for this if you do it at work. You will need a fridge or coolbag to store the milk. Use the coolbag to get the milk home, too. You should also have the means to sterilize any expressing equipment you need. You will probably need to express at home as well, if you are fully breastfeeding.

There are countries where mothers are allowed nursing breaks. If your baby is nearby, this means you can go to feed him, which is probably a lot more convenient than trying to find a place to express and store your milk.

WEEKENDS AND HOLIDAYS

You can fully breastfeed or breastfeed more often when you are away from work and with your baby. This may cause some 'disruption' in your breasts, which will sometimes produce a lot of milk and sometimes not. But usually it's no more than a feeling of fullness, which you'll need to deal with by expressing on your days back at work.

5

STOPPING BREASTFEEDING

It needn't be difficult or distressing for either you or your baby to stop breastfeeding – if that's what you want to do.

If you're stopping before you really want to, turn to pages 108–110, since the situation is then made much more complex by physical and emotional aspects.

BEFORE SIX MONTHS

If you're fully breastfeeding, or mainly breastfeeding, and you want to change over to fully or mainly bottle feeding, aim to drop one breast feed every few days and substitute a bottle feed (see pages 90–91). A useful rule of thumb is to think of taking a fortnight to make the complete switch.

If you go more quickly than this, you may end up with full, uncomfortable breasts, which could lead to blocked ducts and mastitis (see pages 70–71).

BEFORE A YEAR

Most mothers find the last feeds to go are the morning and the evening feed, plus feeds during the night. You can continue with these, or even just one feed, for a long time, even indefinitely, if your baby is around a year old. Trying to get down to one or two feeds a day is not usually as successful with a baby who's a bit younger – the production line seems to need longer before it becomes sufficiently reliable and resilient.

Work out the times of the day at which your baby is least interested in a breastfeed. When you would normally offer one, or you'd expect him to ask, try a cup, a snack or some sort of distraction.

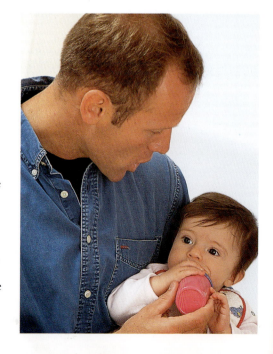

Sometimes, a baby likes a feed to help him settle down for a daytime nap. Instead, you might need to put him into the car for a ride, or take him for a trip in the pram or pushchair. This is probably kinder and gentler than just cuddling, or putting him down to sleep without a feed.

You don't need to teach your baby how to use a bottle after this time, since he is old enough to get the fluid he needs from a cup.

5

A BABY OLDER THAN A YEAR

Once your baby gets into toddlerhood, he may start asking for feeds, and become more pro-active – climbing on to your lap and lifting your top, for instance. This is fine, but if your idea is to stop breastfeeding, not to make it even more popular with your child, you may have to make a decision to stick to one or two feeds at the same time each day, in order to help your child learn what to expect.

STOPPING THE LAST FEEDS

If you do this very gradually, by being already up and about when the early morning feed normally happens (even if it's very early) and having someone else put your child to bed from time to time, you will be able to reduce your breastfeeds slowly and gently.

If at first your child seems distressed by not being allowed to breastfeed and can't be distracted, then just feed him – it is not worth fighting over, and you can always try again tomorrow.

But if you have made a clear decision to stop completely, then it's not fair sometimes to feed, sometimes to feed after a struggle, and sometimes to stick to your guns and refuse. Your child may learn that you can be manipulated by a prolonged whining session – and breastfeeding will begin to be something you start to share with him only resentfully.

5

THE OLDER TODDLER

You can negotiate with children aged two or three. They can learn that 'later' or 'not now' doesn't mean 'no, not ever', and they can learn to wait without getting desperate. Partial weaning can, therefore, sometimes be easier at this age.

If you get to the stage where you want to stop completely, tell your child. You can say that some things are for little boys and girls and not for bigger ones. Work on reducing the feeds to a minimum – one mother installed a wall telephone and used this instead of a phone near the sofa, since her daughter always regarded her mother sitting down to answer the telephone as a reminder to feed.

By this age, you'll know what works with your child. You're cleverer than he is, and you can keep one step ahead.

NIGHTTIME FEEDS

Breastfeeding is often an excellent way to get a wakeful toddler back to sleep. Families who co-sleep find their breastfeeding older baby learns to help himself – and that pattern can continue for a long time.

If your child is in a bed or a cot and wakes at night, or if you want to teach him to stay asleep in a cot and not share with you, but he will only settle with a breastfeed, you can use sleep training to break the habit. Ask your health visitor for support to get this established.

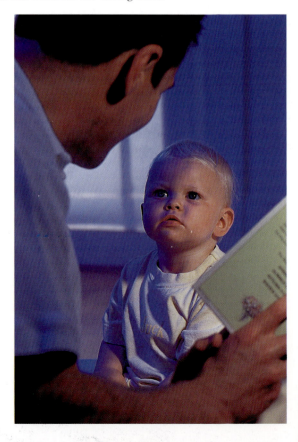

The basic method is to settle your child with the minimum soothing necessary, without taking him out of the bed or cot (and without feeding him). Always respond to his cries, but reassure him, and then leave.

It can take a few nights to achieve a result with this method, but it works if you feel confident and stick with it.

5

GETTING STARTED

■ Get professional help with positioning and attachment. Experiment. You may find it more comfortable to feed both babies at once, or one at a time.

■ Be prepared to change – the position that worked an hour ago, or yesterday, may not work today.

■ Think about your choice of positioning when feeding both together. Decide which works best: one baby under each arm; legs towards legs; or legs pointing in the same direction so that one baby is across you and one is under your arm.

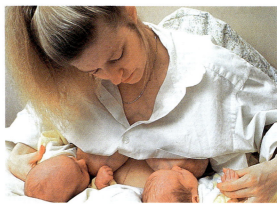

■ Use pillows to help in the early days, since you won't have a spare hand to help with positioning.

■ Try to work out which baby is the better sucker – there's usually one who is a keener and more effective feeder than her sibling – and alternate breasts and babies at each feed. That way you ensure that the poorer sucker gets the chance to take advantage of the stimulation brought about by the other baby.

■ If you have time, express. Then, if you need to accept an offer of help, you have expressed breast milk to give, in a bottle or cup, instead of formula.

FEEDING TRIPLETS

It's harder to breastfeed triplets, after all you have only two breasts. The feeding production line is that much more difficult – and the babies are even more likely to be pre-term or small. It is possible to breastfeed triplets fully, although mothers may have to introduce a bottle of expressed breast milk (or formula) occasionally, and even routinely, with someone else helping out. There are just not enough hours in the day otherwise. You also need to be careful to remember which babies have had a 'turn' on the breast.

TALK TO OTHER PARENTS

Parents are the greatest source of information and support regarding feeding, since their personal experience of looking after more than one baby will have taught them far more than you can learn here, or from health professionals.

There is probably a twins and multiples support group in your area – ask your midwife or health visitor for information.

YOUR PRE-TERM BABY

Babies develop their sucking and swallowing reflexes after about 34 to 35 weeks of pregnancy. A baby born before this time will, therefore, not be able to suck at the breast and will have to get her nutrition in some other way, usually through a tube.

Very tiny newborns – those born at 25 to 28 weeks of pregnancy – are especially vulnerable, and they face several months in special or intensive care. All pre-term babies are at risk of having health problems with their breathing and digestion, or infection, but generally speaking, the smaller and earlier your baby is, the greater her need for specialized care.

THE IMPORTANCE OF BREAST MILK

Your pre-term baby's paediatrician is likely to encourage you to give her breast milk. It's been shown to improve the survival rates of small babies and to protect them against infection.

You can start expressing, by hand at first, to get colostrum for your baby. It's probably not a good idea to use the pump initially, since the amounts of milk are so small that they can stick on the inside of the pump's tubing.

You should maintain regular expressing and, after the volume of your milk has increased, start using an electric pump if you prefer. If you are still in hopsital with your baby, the midwives will help you to learn how to express efficiently. The milk can be given to your baby via a tube. The medical team may feel she needs additional calories, and some supplementary formula specially prepared for pre-term babies may be given.

The best way to feed tiny babies is still under research – after all, it's only in the last few years that babies as young as 25 weeks have had any hope of survival. It is known that breast milk is valuable, however, and that the mother's pre-term milk seems especially suitable. Yet babies do grow better with additional formula, and this is thought to be helpful in mimicking the growth of the baby in the uterus.

But giving your pre-term baby formula should not affect your ability to breastfeed her exclusively when she is able to come to your breast.

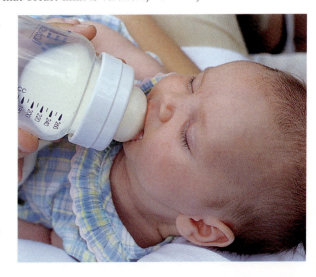

6

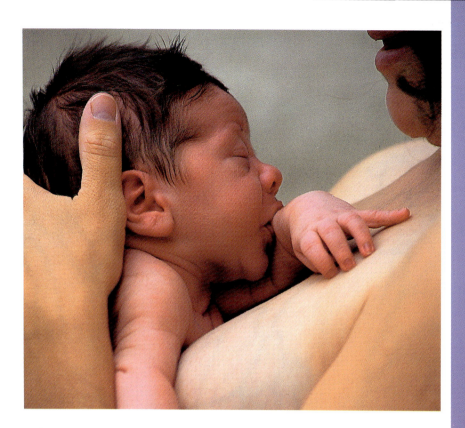

HOLD YOUR BABY WHEN YOU CAN

When your baby is well enough, you can take her out of her incubator, and hold her next to you, tucked into your chest, giving 'kangaroo cuddles' or 'kangaroo care' – perhaps for just a few minutes at a time at first. Be guided by the medical and nursing staff. This is good for later breastfeeding – the smell and feel of your skin will become familiar to her.

You can hold her near your breast and let her lick the nipple and enjoy the taste of it. She may not be able to suck on it yet, but stimulating her reflexes and giving her some practice in just being there is very valuable.

AS YOUR BABY GETS BIGGER...

As she learns to suck and swallow, your baby's time on the breast can be increased. This can be a difficult period for you, and you will need a lot of patience and dedication. Your baby will take quite some time to learn about breastfeeding, and while she's doing so, she will continue to need your expressed breast milk in a tiny cup or a bottle, or via the tube.

Your baby will probably need to be woken for feeds for some weeks, even after she leaves special care. Take it as a sign of health and energy when she starts to be alert and eager for feeds and is feeding often – don't think it means you aren't making enough milk for her.

6

SPECIAL NEEDS BABIES

If you're told your baby has a learning difficulty, or a disability, or a serious congenital problem, such as a heart defect that may need major treatment at some stage, it's natural to feel shock, powerlessness and huge anxiety.

These feeling aren't conducive to happy breastfeeding, but if you had planned to breastfeed, you can still do so.

Ask your doctor, health visitor or midwife if you can speak to another health professional with special knowledge, or to a parent who has had experience of feeding a baby with the same problem as yours.

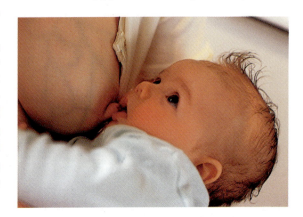

POOR FEEDERS

Breastfeeding supporters have almost all seen or heard of babies who fail to grow, and where the health professionals have all assumed a breastfeeding problem – probably undersupply. Yet when the baby is switched to formula, the same situation occurs. The baby is just not very interested. Then, further tests reveal an underlying health problem and, by that time, the breastfeeding may be lost.

BABIES WITH HEART DEFECTS

A baby who feeds poorly, who doesn't gain weight, and who seems to have difficulty coordinating her sucking, may have an undiagnosed congenital problem. For instance, this could be an indication of a baby who is suffering from a heart defect.

She may manage to take enough breast milk to 'tick over' and to prevent dehydration, but all her energy is being used up in surviving – and she has none left over to suck for longer or, more often, to grow.

Heart problems are not always diagnosed at birth, and it is always worthwhile getting a specialist's advice if your baby fails to thrive.

BABIES WITH DEVELOPMENTAL DELAY

It can be difficult to diagnose the extent of developmental delay, but when feeding problems persist, it is something doctors will want to check for, alongside other investigations.

6

DOWN'S SYNDROME BABIES

Babies born with Down's syndrome have a special problem with sucking. The tongue tends to push the breast out of the mouth. If your baby has difficulty in keeping the breast in her mouth because of this, occupational therapists can sometimes help.

You can also try different positions, in the hope that finding the right one will encourage your baby to learn 'better' sucking. It may be that a bottle is the only truly effective way of getting the milk into her. Some Down's babies do, however, manage to breastfeed very well, either directly or via a bottle.

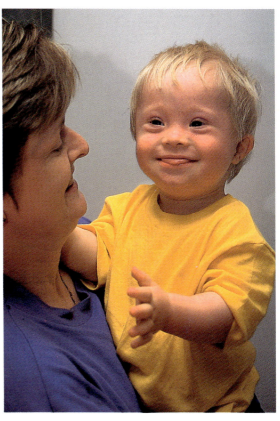

If your Down's baby needs surgery at a later stage – because of a heart problem, which tends to be more common in these babies – your breast milk may be especially important in building up her resistance to infection.

CLEFT LIP OR PALATE

Babies are occasionally born with a gap in their palate and/or upper lip, on one or both sides of the face.

Skilled surgery means that the gap can be closed, but this may not take place for some months. In the meantime, your baby needs to feed – and sometimes it is not possible for her to make an adequate seal on the breast so that she can feed.

If your baby can't feed at the breast, you can express and feed her with a special feeder bottle which closes off the palate, to prevent the milk coming back down through the nose. Some surgeons give cleft lip-and-palate babies a protective shield which they wear instead.

Discuss the details of feeding with your doctor, and ask to talk to other mothers who have breastfed babies with this condition. They may well have useful tips for you.

Again, since your baby will need corrective surgery at some point, breast milk is important to help build up resistance to infection.

6

WHEN YOUR BABY IS ILL

If your baby becomes ill, then breastfeeding may be the only form of nourishment she's willing to take, even if she has been used to solid food alongside her breastfeeds.

There is normally no reason to stop breastfeeding your baby, although if she needs surgery you should take advice from medical staff about when to offer the last feed before she is anaesthetized.

It used to be thought that babies with diarrhoea and vomiting should be taken off milk, including breast milk, and given water or rehydrating fluids instead. Now, this advice has been superseded by the knowledge that breast milk is not only well tolerated by a sick baby, but actively speeds recovery.

YOUR BABY IN HOSPITAL

Stay with your baby as much as you can if she needs hospital care, and continue to breastfeed her. The evidence is that babies and young children actually recover more quickly if they can have the comfort of being close to a parent in such unfamiliar and frightening surroundings. If you have to be separated for any reason, maintain your milk supply by expressing.

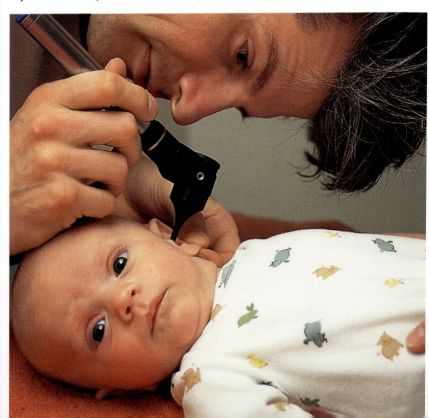

YOUR BABY'S NAPPIES

A fully breastfed baby is very unlikely to suffer from constipation or diarrhoea. Nevertheless, mothers (and even some doctors) worry that this may be the case, but be reassured.

■ It is normal, after the first weeks, for a baby to go several days between bowel movements. She is not suffering from constipation if she shows this pattern. It is also normal for her motions to be quite frequent. Anything in between is also acceptable, as long as your baby is healthy and thriving.

■ It is normal for your baby's motions to be soft. She does not have diarrhoea if her stools are soft and yellow – that's the usual colour of the stools of a fully breastfed baby. Diarrhoea is rare in a fully breastfed baby. It shows as mucousy, watery stools, and your baby may be vomiting, and appear feverish and weak.

■ The occasional green stool is also common. In a healthy, thriving baby it is not significant; it just means her milk has been digested very quickly for some reason.

■ Frothy, mucousy stools can sometimes be an indication that you need to let your baby stay on the first breast for as long as she wants to. It has been suggested that these stools are a symptom of too much fore milk, so allowing your baby to come off the first side only when she wants to helps her take the hind milk she needs.

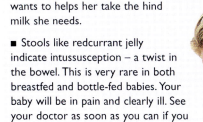

■ Stools like redcurrant jelly indicate intussusception – a twist in the bowel. This is very rare in both breastfed and bottle-fed babies. Your baby will be in pain and clearly ill. See your doctor as soon as you can if you suspect your baby is suffering from diarrhoea or intussusception.

TAKING MEDICATION

While it's sensible to be cautious about any medication you are prescribed when you are breastfeeding, there's no need to worry that everything and anything you take can get into your milk.

Some drugs simply don't reach the milk at all. Others may reach it, but they can't harm the baby because they are not absorbable by the gut – and that includes the baby's gut. Some drugs may reach the breast milk, be absorbed by the baby and have no harmful effect. Some drugs may reach the breast milk in such tiny quantities that the experts are not concerned about it.

If you need to take medication, then tell or remind your doctor that you are breastfeeding. If you want something without prescription, check with the pharmacist.

In many instances, any contraindications are there because tests have not yet been done to 'clear' the drug. In almost every case, a drug which is contraindicated during breastfeeding can be replaced with one that's known to be safe. Alternatively, perhaps you could wait until your baby is older and taking less breast milk before taking the drug.

There is hardly ever any overwhelming need to wean your baby from the breast if you have to take medication.

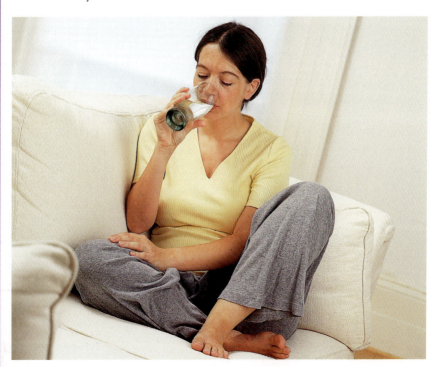

DRUGS ABOUT WHICH THERE IS CONCERN

Certain drugs are not compatible with breastfeeding. These include some of the major tranquillizers such as Librium, which is only ever prescribed to mothers who are severely mentally ill, perhaps with the most serious form of post-natal illness known as puerperal psychosis.

Some doctors are also concerned about the use of other drugs used to treat depression such as Prozac, which is generally not advised for breastfeeding mothers. But discuss this with your doctor, information may change as knowledge increases.

Drugs to control epilepsy are not considered safe for the baby receiving breast milk – but even here, dosages can be timed, and feeds scheduled, to 'dodge' the time when the drug might appear in the milk. Having to do this makes it much less easy to breastfeed as often as your baby wants, and you may occasionally need to express and discard your milk, or give expressed breast milk collected when you know your milk is drug-free.

This list of drugs to avoid is by no means exhaustive. Always discuss your needs, and your baby's needs, with your doctor. In very rare cases, you may be advised to express and discard your milk. This is known as 'pump and dump'.

ANTIBIOTICS

Some antibiotics are more widely prescribed for breastfeeding mothers than others because they are known to be safe. Some mothers say their babies have looser stools after they themselves have been taking antibiotics, but this is nothing to worry about.

CAN ILLNESS PREVENT BREASTFEEDING?

In the West, mothers who are HIV positive are currently advised not to breastfeed, since it is thought that the baby may contract HIV through the milk. This is a real risk, although statistics are inconclusive.

Mothers with all forms of hepatitis need to take up-to-date advice, but currently it's considered safe for them to breastfeed.

If you are ill with flu or some other non-serious illness, don't stop breastfeeding. Your body is already producing the antibodies to that illness and your baby needs them in your breast milk. It makes no sense to stay away from her to avoid passing on your germs – stay close and you'll pass on the immunities to her.

LONG-TERM MEDICATION

If you have a chronic condition, such as diabetes or asthma, it should still be possible to breastfeed and continue with your normal medication. Ask you doctor about this.

Remember: breastfeeding reduces the risk of your baby developing several conditions, including both of these illnesses.

6

CONTRACEPTION

Most women find that their periods are delayed when they are breastfeeding. This is normal, and it's a reaction to the hormonal changes that take place as breastfeeding gets under way.

Some women find their periods don't return for a long time after the birth of their baby, maybe not until after breastfeeding stops completely, although it's more common for them to return when breastfeeding is less frequent, or is supplemented with other foods. They may return if your baby stops feeding during the night.

CONTRACEPTIVES TO USE WHEN BREASTFEEDING

Methods advised

Contraceptive pill	Progesterone only pill has low levels of hormones which do not affect the milk supply.
Condom	Fully effective
Cap, or diaphragm	Get your existing one checked for size after the birth; it may need to be changed.
Gel or cream	Safe to use with condom or cap during breastfeeding.
Coil or IUCD	Get it inserted at a clinic or by your doctor at or after the six-week post-natal check.

Methods not advised

Combined pill	Contains progesterone, testosterone and oestrogen, which tends to reduce the milk supply.
Injections	Contraceptive injections also contain oestrogen and so may reduce the milk supply.

CAN BREASTFEEDING ACT AS A CONTRACEPTIVE?

Breastfeeding is the most widely used form of child-spacing in the world. If you are not menstruating and are feeding your baby several times during both the day and the night, your contraceptive protection is as high as that given by the pill, according to research.

But in the West, very few mothers breastfeed as often as that. We try to prolong the gaps between feeds, and we are more likely to introduce other fluids and other foods than mothers in the developing world.

This is why family planning experts advocate the 'lactational amenorrhoea method' (the method using the lack of periods associated with breastfeeding) only to mothers who are committed to it and who understand it. But it's certainly a safe method, with no side effects.

It can be effective for longer than six months if you combine it with watching for symptoms of ovulation (by checking cervical mucus), and by not having penetrative sex at a time when you think you may be fertile.

BREASTFEEDING WHEN YOU ARE PREGNANT

It is, of course, possible to become pregnant while you are breastfeeding, and indeed you may want to have another child quickly.

If you want to continue feeding, that's fine. There is no good reason to stop. When your new baby is born you will produce colostrum as normal, then your milk will come in, just as it would if you had not been breastfeeding. Sometimes the first child goes off the breast at this time, then comes back to it once more.

Feeding a baby and a toddler, or child, is called 'tandem feeding'. It's usually advised that you should let the new baby feed first, especially when she is very young. Later you can feed both children together.

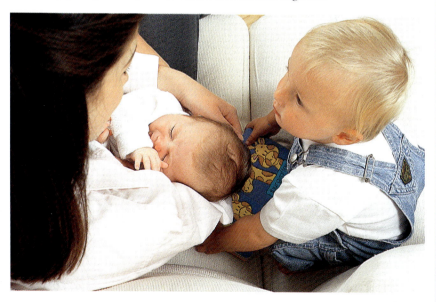

IF IT ISN'T WORKING

If you decide to give up breastfeeding, or exclusive breastfeeding, even if you had planned to do it for a lot longer, you're bound to have mixed emotions. which you won't want to share with people who try to tell you it doesn't really matter. These emotions could include:

■ Regret and disappointment – because you have tried hard to make a success of breastfeeding.

■ Guilt – because you think you have failed your baby, yet feel liberated from the struggle of it all and, in turn, feel bad at reacting that way.

■ Anger – because you may think you have not had sufficient help to make a success of breastfeeding and that your body has let you down.

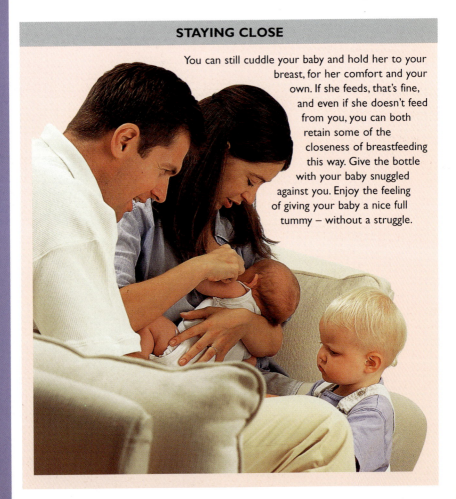

STAYING CLOSE

You can still cuddle your baby and hold her to your breast, for her comfort and your own. If she feeds, that's fine, and even if she doesn't feed from you, you can both retain some of the closeness of breastfeeding this way. Give the bottle with your baby snuggled against you. Enjoy the feeling of giving your baby a nice full tummy – without a struggle.

YOUR FEELINGS

It's normal to have different emotions – positive and negative – all these feelings are understandable. Breastfeeding is more than just a way of getting milk into babies. It's a relationship – with your baby, of course, but also with your own body.

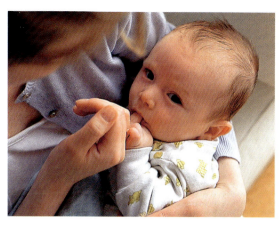

■ If breastfeeding hasn't gone well, you can feel let down by your body – angry and frustrated by it, puzzled and confused.

■ If you think you haven't had the right support and information about how to make breastfeeding suit you and your baby, or if you've been given conflicting advice that leaves you wondering which way to turn, you may feel angry with yourself and with those you relied on for the right sort of care.

■ You could even feel embarrassed at being seen giving your baby a bottle in public – the opposite of the awkwardness some women feel at breastfeeding in front of others.

Yet if things have gone badly, or painfully, or you have lost confidence in breastfeeding – for whatever reason – switching to the bottle may be a relief. At least it's one thing you do not have to battle with any longer.

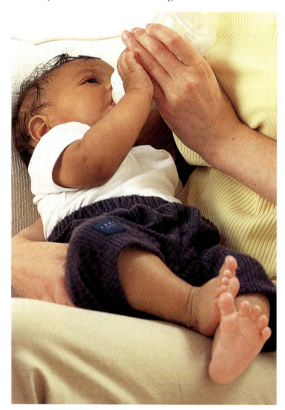

THE EASIEST WAY TO GIVE UP

Don't stop suddenly. Reduce your milk supply gradually. This may already be happening if you're giving formula, but formalize it by giving a top-up of formula after most feeds and then every feed, or by substituting formula for one extra breastfeed every few days.

If you have been breastfeeding for only a few weeks – less than six, say – you can go a little faster than this. Just make sure you don't get engorged and watch for any lumps in your breasts, indicating blocked ducts or mastitis.

THE AFTERMATH

If you have to give up beastfeeding, it's easy to have a long-lasting resentment of any mention of 'breast is best'. Women who do manage to breastfeed longer than you do seem smug and self-satisfied, and you may even think they're being critical of you for not 'sticking with it'.

Here's how to feel more positive about the situation.

■ Accept that there are many things we plan for our children that don't work out, and that feeding intention is just one of them.

■ Try to understand what went wrong – there's almost always an explanation for breastfeeding problems.

■ Stop blaming yourself. You tried, it didn't work, you didn't get the right help – it wasn't your fault.

■ Feel good about the breastfeeding you did do.

■ Look forward, not back, to a time when your biggest food-related worry will be how to get mashed potato and gravy stains out of your best blouse.

■ Accept that while formula milk is not the same as breast milk, and breast milk is undoubtedly superior in many ways, formula has made several steps forward from the substitutes given to babies even 10 years ago.

■ Don't apologise for bottle feeding. People are not nearly as critical as you imagine they are when your feelings are raw.

■ Remind yourself that feeding is not the be-all and end-all of mothering, just one part of it, and only you can judge when and if the negatives of breastfeeding outweigh the positives.

■ Allow yourself to grieve if you feel sad about it. Those people who say, 'It doesn't matter', can be forgiven because they really don't understand.

■ Above all, remember that even if things have not worked out this time, you may have the chance to try again with another baby, when you will be able to seek the right help and support from the start and, by drawing on your present experience, to establish successful breastfeeding without the struggle you have had this time.

CAN I START AGAIN?

It's perfectly possible to start breastfeeding again after a period without either feeding your baby or expressing milk. This is known as relactation, and you can relactate at any stage as long as you have a cooperative baby.

RELACTATING

It is easier to induce your milk to return if:

■ it's only been a short time since you stopped breastfeeding – days or weeks rather than months – and you had established a good supply of milk before you stopped.

■ your baby is happy to come to the breast and suckle, even if she doesn't get rewarded with a lot, or even any, milk.

■ you express milk with a pump or by hand at least every few hours.

■ you express or feed your baby during the night.

Just try it! Put your baby to the breast and see what her reaction is. The more you can do this, the more likely it is you can bring your milk back. You can gradually reduce the formula she's having as your milk returns. But be aware that it may not work if your baby has forgotten what to do, or if she associates the breast with a struggle.

BREASTFEEDING WITHOUT PREGNANCY

Some mothers have induced breast milk for adopted babies even without being pregnant, although a full milk supply is never likely, and they need to be very consistent and motivated. These mothers usually use expressing – there will be nothing to express at first – plus a nursing supplementer. This is a small bag of formula worn between the breasts at feed time. It is attached to a tube, the end of which is taped to the nipple. The baby sucks at the nipple – which stimulates lactation – and gets formula, which rewards her for sucking.

6

INDEX

ACKNOWLEDGEMENTS

The author and the publishers gratefully acknowledge the invaluable contribution made by
Adrian Weinbrecht who took all the photographs in this book except:
pp. 38, 99, 101, 102, Angela Hampton. pp. 39, 62, 97 Anthea Sieveking.
The illustrations were produced by Sheilagh Noble and Kuo Kang Chen.